'BYE T2D

'BYE T2D

DEFEATING DIABETES

G. Sreeprakash

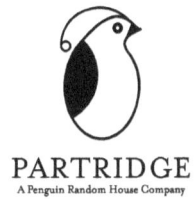

PARTRIDGE

A Penguin Random House Company

To order additional copies of this book, contact
Partridge India
000 800 10062 62
www.partridgepublishing.com/india
orders.india@partridgepublishing.com

CONTENTS

To all those who would like to keep diabetes at arm's length.

1 'BYE T2D

What prompted me to write these experiences of mine is the gross inadequacy of required information available on Type 2 Diabetes to a large cross section of the population across the globe. It is a matter of concern for every one that the number of persons affected by diabetes is increasing rapidly all over the place. The sheer economic burden of providing effective medical care to all these persons is growing day by day with serious economic consequences for nations in the years to come. In order that matters related to this are put in the correct perspective, an attempt is made to educate people at large about this.

Diabetes needs to be brought into the domain of serious health hazards for a growing number of persons all across the world. Diabetes is essentially a life style disorder playing havoc with one's metabolism and in the process opening the gateway to a wide range of serous diseases. It complicates the management of just about all matters related to one's health. If one is free from Type 2 Diabetes, all conditions warranting health care will become much more manageable and amenable to cure. The condition needs to be effectively addressed through a combination of dietary changes, life style changes with focus on engaging in appropriate physical activity on a regular basis and administering appropriate drugs including insulin injections where required. But unfortunately this seems to have been not properly registered with most persons including the affected persons and sometimes even with the medical practitioners themselves. The role of self management in diabetes is very important and its significance can not be ignored. As a matter of fact self management forms over two thirds of management as far as diabetes is concerned. The role of external management obviously is not as important as that of self management.

Diabetes is not an illness in the sense that it is not like having a fever which subsides on taking of paracetamol. Far from that it needs a multi-pronged approach largely falling in the domain of self management. People who are just dependent on medicines with no concern for the other two equally if not more important aspects—dietary changes and appropriate physical activity—are seen to extensively suffer from and fall victims to their perverted perceptions about the condition that diabetes unfortunately brings with it. As a case in point, I know of a number of cases of persons who pass off while engaged in walking or otherwise engaging in physical activities as directed by physicians. Physicians prescribe medicines and recommend reduced intake of food and increased physical activity as a kind of routine and default prescription for people seeing them with request for treatment of sugar control. The number of persons who pass off on account of promptly and religiously taking medicines and refraining from eating as required of them and engaging in walking or mild exercise is seen to increase with every passing day with many of them falling prey to severe hypoglycemia leading to collapse and in very many cases to untimely, unfortunate and avoidable death. I had wondered if only they were a little better educated about diabetes. The point is when there is more physical activity you need either more food intake and/or lower medication. Likewise when there is less food intake, you need to avoid unnecessary physical activity. Medicinal intake should be suited to the context of the combination of one's physical activity and food intake. Similarly when you indulge in eating more food for whatever reason, you require more medicine. These things can be put to practice only when one has a proper awareness about the condition that leads to diabetes.

While taking medicines as prescribed is generally welcome like eating light and doing exercise, one should be aware of the overall effect of a dynamic combination of these factors to appreciate and effectively manage diabetes in the manner it is to be managed.

2 OH! THOSE DAYS

I could not believe it. Never in my wildest thoughts did I imagine that I would be free from the clutches of this dreaded disease. I had heard so much about the illness that every one I discussed the matter with was mentioning that I would be a slave to this disease for the rest of my life.

What was worrisome was that this included some of my doctor friends as well. Some of them were having diabetes for some length of time as well. They were all swearing that once you contract this disease, there is no getting out of it. Even people close to me who always wanted to be and painstakingly practised to be positive about every thing were hopelessly maintaining that any one who gets this disease will be married to it for the rest of his life.

Not just me. Any one diagnosed as having diabetes will remain that way. People including medical practitioners of all shades used to maintain that one can only manage the disease but can not get over it.

But here I am testing negative for high blood sugar for the twelfth month in a row. For the fourth time the three-month test being carried out technically referred to as A1C has shown a value just below six. This by all accounts is a confirmation that I am no longer a diabetic. In fact I on my own was conducting blood test off and on using a glucometer with blood collected at various points of time of the day spread over months. Fasting, post-breakfast, post-lunch, post-dinner, random and what not—a hundred different readings all confirmed that my blood sugar levels were always within permissible limits.

Sceptical doctors who could not believe it insisted on my conducting the special test that is carried out every three months which gives the average blood sugar value for the three month period or so. That is the test referred to as A1C. This is supposed to give the average for a three-to-four month period and is considered as the most dependable test of blood sugar over a period of time. This is supposed to be very accurate and the test for the fourth time in a row has proved conclusively that I was not a diabetic any more.

At the end of eleven years after having tested positive for diabetes, here I am free of that illness. Even I could not believe it.

3 DIABETES—WHAT IS IT?

I had not seen my grandfather. I was told that my grandfather was a leading lawyer and public figure in that locality. Despite being a busy lawyer he could devote time for extensive social work and could attend to spiritual discourses as well. He had been by all accounts a very busy person.

Grandfather passed away when he was fifty five years of age. I was not even born then. From what people used to say he suffered from no illness other than diabetes. The immediate reason for his death was some swellings on his back which refused to go away. In relation to its treatment by way of elementary surgical intervention he had to be hospitalized for a week or so. He unfortunately never returned from that hospital.

Such was the picture I had of diabetes. I used to think of it as some kind of a diabolic illness which unkindly took away my grandfather who in my view then did not have to leave that soon. At least before seeing me. Diabetes for me was a dreaded disease resulting in untimely and premature death. This attitude got hardened inside me by the way my mother used to say once in a while about diabetes. Whenever test was conducted to rule out high blood sugar, she used to mention that she would not like to live long in case she was diagnosed with diabetes. Those days urine test was done once in a while and blood test for diabetes detection used to be rather infrequent.

Talking about tests being conducted, regular blood check started being done properly only in the eighties or so. I was amazed to know that in slightly older times diabetes test was conducted with urine poured around ant hills. If ants gathered around the urinated area one was detected positive for diabetes; if not one was considered as detected negative for diabetes.

Things have moved forward quite a bit from those days. Now we know that only after sugar is found in excess of permissible levels in the blood only sugar begins to appear in urine. As a consequence of this, not having sugar traces in urine is not conclusive proof of one being a non-diabetic. That is to say all diabetics need not have traces of sugar present in their urine. But having sugar traces in urine is definitely an indicator that one is having diabetes, and not only that—the blood sugar level is probably worrisomely high.

All these things I was aware of because of my being a rather prolific reader of just about anything in print including books and magazines of all kinds. Just like my grandfather, I used to articulate my views on matters including illness in any group I could find myself being in. I enjoyed discussing matters of interest with friends and colleagues. In fact persons in my circle of friends used to enjoy this—at least that was the feeling I used to get.

It is during such discussions that I got acquainted with the treatment for diabetes in *Ayurveda* the ancient Indian science of longevity. Ayurveda deals at length with the state of having diabetes variously referred to as *madhumeha* and *prameha* among others. As per Ayurveda I came to understand that there are twenty different types of *meha* associated with the imbalance of *vata, pitta* and *kapha*, the *tridoshas*. (Loosely translated kapha stands for matter, vatha for energy and pitta the process of converting matter into energy. Persons who have an excess of kapha or matter not getting converted into energy are prone to getting diabetes). Ayurveda holds prameha as exhibiting the symptom of getting tired for no particular reason. It is said: If you feel like walking while you want to run, if you feel like sitting while you want to walk, if you feel like lying down while you want to sit, and if you feel like sleeping while you want to lie down, in the ordinary course of your day to day activities, you have diabetes.

Clinically however matters are not as simple as this. Now I know that the most accepted indication of having diabetes is to have blood sugar going beyond permissible levels. The permissible levels are 80 to 110 mg/dL at fasting or before meals, less than 160 mg/dL two hours after meals and 100 to 140 mg/dL at bed time. In case of values above this, one is variously referred to as having a pre-diabetic condition or diabetic depending on how much the sugar levels are in excess of these levels. So also there is a blood test being carried out at three-monthly intervals referred to as HbA1C or simply A1C in which if the reading is above 6 % it represents a diabetic condition.

Diabetes is caused by either lack of insulin or insulin resistance. Diabetes is classified in clinical medicine into three. They are Type 1 Diabetes or T 1 D which is characterized by a total lack of insulin from the pancreas. Type 2 Diabetes or T2D is generally found with advancing age and is brought about by the inability of pancreas to secrete the required amounts of insulin or inadequacy in the insulin carrying system of the body or a combination of both. Then there is what is referred to as gestational diabetes which is blood sugar spiking of a temporary nature like the spiking of blood sugar levels associated with pregnancies in certain cases. However a vast majority of cases fall under T2D and that is the condition we are discussing here.

T2D is the most prevalent form of diabetes. The onset of T2D used to be at ages well beyond the middle age earlier on. For example, about fifty years ago it was very difficult to locate a diabetic aged below fifty years of age. But over the years for various reasons the picture has been taking a turn for the worse with a very large number of persons below the age of forty being tested positive for Type 2 Diabetes. What is more unfortunate is that most diabetics below forty years—for that matter diabetics who are fifty years or more of age as well—are not even aware of their blood sugar levels being far above the permissible levels.

Essentially T2D sets in when insulin secretion from the beta cells of the pancreas fails to maintain blood glucose levels within the permissible limits. Type 2 Diabetes can simply be stated as accelerated ageing with attendant debilitating effects on just about every system in the body. Over the years, left unattended and unmanaged, it results in life threatening complications related to cardiovascular functioning, degeneration of the nervous system, kidney dysfunction, retinal problems leading to blindness, erectile dysfunction and a steep decline in the quality of one's life all around.

Like hypertension, T2D is in a way a silent killer. Very few symptoms of T2D manifest till it is very late the progression of the condition. In fact T2D is very often diagnosed as part of blood test conducted in connection with some other condition as part of routine check up. Even when diagnosed it is unfortunate that very few people give required attention to this and just wish away sanguine in the feeling that 'I have got some sugar problem, it's nothing much' kind of disdain. This indeed is very pathetic and is an indication of how poorly diabetic literate are the people at large. Apart from being a very serious condition very likely to bring with it all possible complications with regard to one's health, the economic aspect of taking care of this condition from slipping into dangerous zones is very alarming. As of now T2D is the major contributor to blindness, kidney failure and heart failure with advancing age.

Insulin secreted by pancreas is required by cells for carrying glucose from the food to the tissues in the body. When the secretion level of insulin is low or when the carrying capacity of the cells is impaired on account of any reason glucose is not absorbed by the tissues requiring it. The unabsorbed glucose as it is then gets into the blood stream thus increasing the blood sugar levels. Capacity of the pancreas to secrete insulin diminishes with advancing age and just on account of this the possibility of one developing T2D increases as one gets older. This is one reason why one needs to settle down for a lower food intake with advancing age. If food intake is maintained undiminished as one gets old, the development of getting T2D gets that much accelerated. Inadequate carrying capacity is brought about by accumulation of fat in and around the stomach area referred to in medical world as central obesity or Syndrome X. Central obesity is in fact the most common reason, central obesity being the accumulation of fat in the stomach area. This development seriously hampers the carrying capacity of cells thus resulting in less and less of insulin really reaching the tissues. Looked at from another angle, the impaired carrying capacity results in the requirement of larger amounts of insulin to be carried to deliver a given amount of glucose to the tissues. This further accelerates the decline in the capacity of pancreas to secrete insulin. This can be thought of as something like the pancreas having a definite stock of insulin which it secretes over its life cycle in full. The early heavy drain in this results in something like the pancreas running out of insulin faster than it normally should. This is not exactly the position, but is being put so to make the understanding clear. This excessive use of insulin is referred to as insulin resistance. This is what results in obese people with central obesity who seldom engage in physical activity and who keep on eating the wrong kind of food keep on showing normal blood sugar values for some time. Little do they realize that they are proceeding rapidly down the track of developing T2D.

Overeating and sedentary life style are the two contributors to one developing central obesity and thus insulin resistance. In fact sedentary life generally follows overeating. Eating more than the normal requirement of food makes one feel lethargic and makes one burdened with increased weight to be carried around. So also, it is heavily taxing one's metabolic apparatus by feeding it with more food to work on. Any which way one looks at it, it is a pathetic situation leading one down the undesirable path of ill health.

Blood sugar levels are maintained to be normal if they are maintained between 80 to 110 mg/dL at fasting or before meals; less than 170 mg/dL about two hours after meals and within 140 mg/dL at bed time. In case of values slightly above this, one is variously referred to as having a pre-diabetic condition or diabetic condition depending on how much the sugar levels are at variance with these levels. Opinions will differ as regards the actual values mentioned above this way or that way a little bit but broadly these levels hold good.

Another test generally carried out every three months indicate a clearer picture of the blood sugar situation over the three month period. This is the HbA1C test popularly mentioned as simply A1C. If the A1C value is above six it indicates a diabetic condition with value beyond six clearly qualifying for confirmation as a diabetic.

4 YOU EAT YOUR WAY INTO T2D

I kept on wondering how sugar levels can get out of range in the case of a person. I knew as well as many others that the human body is an ensemble of very many different components engaged incessantly in the proper completion of millions of processes. These activities are basically directed at ensuring that various parameters are maintained within the permissible levels all by itself. These auto-mechanisms are what in fact keep your body and my body in the shape and condition they are in. That you are reading this sentence and I am writing now is indeed a tribute to the meticulous and harmonious synchronization of these processes. These processes are what contribute to the maintenance of our body temperature irrespective of the temperature outside. These are the processes which ensure that our blood pressure is maintained the way it is. These are the processes which ensure that sodium levels are maintained in a particularly narrow range. These are the processes that help us see, help us walk and so on and so forth. These are again the processes that keep one's blood sugar levels within a healthy range. You can not have a situation where you will have less of sugar come what may. Again you can not have a situation where blood sugar levels are allowed to spike and any which way that wants. Not just blood sugar level, just about every thing associated with the body has to operate within permissible levels. Then how come that one's blood sugar values appear to be on a spiking journey? And worse still, how this anomaly seems to be merrily riding on a path of achieving alarming growth?

This set me on the track of finding out more about how alarming the picture was and also finding out how exactly the body allows increase in blood sugar levels. Metabolism like very many processes associated with the maintenance of body is a very complex process at best only partly understood and worse grossly misquoted about. Globally T2D is assuming alarming proportion as a condition seriously and adversely affecting the quality of life of millions and millions of people in all parts of the world. In India, the situation is even more alarming with its population being what is called 'genetically predisposed to contracting it'. India is also referred to as the emerging diabetic capital of the world.

I began looking around to find out how blood sugar level goes up and stays beyond permissible levels. The gist of what I could understand is given here. It is agreed generally that diabetes is a metabolic disorder and considered that way it is a fact as well as an over simplification of a very complex state of functioning of our body.

Food and Energy

The body needs energy for maintenance of the base level body functions and for carrying out our routine activities related to living. Base level body functions include all activities the body undertakes in maintaining itself like keeping the organs in good condition, repairing of tissues and cells, ensuring that the various systems—the circulatory system, the endocrine system, the nervous system, the skeletal system etc.—are all kept in good shape. Body needs energy for all this. Even while one is fast asleep, the body is working meticulously to ensure that its functions are carried on correctly. For this one needs energy. The energy required for this is referred to as the Base(or Basal) Metabolic Rate or BMR for short.

Over and above BMR you need energy for the conscious self-willed efforts you are putting in. This includes all your physical and mental activities. You need to spend energy for getting up from bed, walking to the toilet, brushing your teeth, bathing, going out in the sun, eating, traveling, performing your official functions, playing, walking so on and so forth. For each and every thing you do you need energy. This is above your BMR requirement.

Now, think for a moment. Where do you get your energy from? From air, sun light and food. Air and sun light is fine.—but modern styles of living severely hampers this also. We will see that later on. However, apart from the marginal input from air and sun light—actually to draw air and to be in sun light you need energy—your most important and major source of energy is food.

One of the most important basic functions of the body is to receive food and convert this into energy. The process of converting food into energy is substantially addressed by your endocrine system. This is where food gets metabolized. Energy is released on proper metabolism of the food you eat. The energy so released is to be passed on to the blood at the cellular level. This is how the food-energy system works. Energy your body can accept at the cellular level only as glucose or sugar in every day language. And cells can accept this energy—that is glucose or sugar—only when it is carried to them by insulin.

Pancreas and Insulin

Pancreas located in our abdominal area is the organ or gland that releases insulin in a healthy individual. More precisely, the beta cells in the pancreas produce insulin. This when released into our digestive system acts as carriers of glucose or sugar into the cells of the body. Unless accompanied by insulin sugar or glucose is not accepted by the body. Food one eats gets converted into glucose which is the only form of energy that the body is required to be constantly supplied with.

In a normal healthy individual pancreas performs the function of releasing as much insulin as is required for digesting the food intake. Like so many amazing things in its maintenance performed by the wonderful mechanism that is our body, pancreas ordinarily releases just about enough insulin required for assimilation of the glucose released into the blood—no less or no more of insulin.

But what happens to the energy being passed on to the cells? This energy is utilized for carrying on the base level bodily functions. These functions—in fact millions and millions of cells carry out the process of rebuilding, repairing and replacing various cells and tissues in our body all the time—are carried on on a steady basis even when you think you are not doing any thing. Whether you think or do not think—even for thinking you need energy—these multifarious activities your body automatically carries out require quite a bit of energy. This is referred to as the base level energy requirement or zero-level energy required for the maintenance of one's basic body functions. A certain amount of energy is required for this and the energy released into the blood stream accompanied or escorted by insulin first takes care of this requirement.

What happens to the rest of the energy released into the blood stream? This is to be utilized for whatever one does other than the automatic bodily functions we referred to above. Energy required by you to walk around, to brush your teeth, to cook your food, to eat it, to drive around, to visit places of interest or friends or just about every thing you consider your activity is to be met out of this. When the aggregate energy you spend on all such activities equals the surplus energy provided by your food all is well.

When the energy you spend is more than the energy you receive by way of food, you feel tired and immediately you reach out for a snack or drink. The deficit in energy is taken care of and made up immediately on your body recognizing it and notifying it. All is fine up to this point.

What about the case of your food intake when it is more than what is required for the energy you expend? This in fact is the case with the vast majority of persons one encounters now. Without being really aware of it, involuntarily people by and large tend to lead sedentary lives with many a bodily function which earlier required physical output on our part now being carried out by technology-enabled devices. Walking is replaced by driving around, drawing and carrying water from well or pond is replaced by water being available on tap, gathering firewood and using it for cooking is replaced by cooking gas available on line, rearing of cows and taking milk from them is replaced by packed milk available from shop shelf and so on and so forth. All these shift in the execution of various tasks has resulted in every one spending much less energy on performing activities which were essential for carrying out our living in the past. Activities human race has been used to for thousands of years are all of a sudden not required to be performed. All activities are virtually reduced to pressing a button in a manner of speaking.

Pressing a button needs a lot less energy than what is required to carry out the processes triggered by the button. The savings in energy is to be utilized else where since we have already got energy available in the form of food taken in and assimilated. This is not a one off case. Always we tend to eat more food than required on a continuous basis on one pretext or other. One does not worry about what happens to the food except that while consuming it tastes good. One finds newer and newer reasons for consuming food—like occasional parties, a birthday splash or celebration, mindless eating indulged in during festive occasions, the exquisite taste of food at this or that restaurant and a hundred different reasons like that. All these, as you can see now, unfortunately imply that your body continuously throws up an unbalanced metabolic equation. The food—read energy—intake is always more than—in fact much much more than—the actual requirement.

What happens to this excess energy? The body has to do some thing about it. It can ill afford to carry it around especially when it is bombarded with more of it on a more or less regular basis. Apart from a portion of such excess energy carried as reserve by liver, the rest is converted into fat and kept at wherever it can be safely kept. Over a period of time this results in your putting on weight. You tend to look fatty, develop a paunch with central obesity setting in, and you obviously look bloated. You tend to be immobile, inactive and even more sedentary on account of this. You become a little vegetable-like.

And this is what essentially takes you through to the road to becoming a diabetic for the rest of your life. Even though there are other factors like heredity, genetic predisposition in respect of certain ethnic groups etc., the single dominant reason for the explosive increase in T2D the world over is the mismatch between the food intake and the activity levels of people. The more alarming aspect of this is that this mismatch has assumed the levels of a cultural phenomenon. The mismatch is not just at the individual level but is very real even at the social level. The mismatch is unfortunately even being treated as a part of the modern culture with partying, fast food joints and irregular, unhealthy eating habits on the increase all the time all over the place. This translates into ill health being courted as a matter of routine. Diabetes unfortunately opens the gateway to all the ailment one comes across, putting all bodily systems completely out of gear over a period of time if allowed a free run. The picture is truly alarming and needs to be addressed with all the might at one's command. And think of it—all this is the result of unbridled, unchecked and unhealthy eating habits.

One eats one's way into T2D.

5 MORE ON FOOD

Talking about food, let us first understand one thing. There is nothing like a food that interacts in the same manner with an individual's metabolism in a given manner at least as far as its impact in a diabetic context is concerned. Foods are classified in terms of the glycemic index to understand their impact as far as blood sugar is concerned. Put simply, glycemic index is an indicator of the time taken by our metabolic system to convert carbohydrate or sugars in a given food into glucose for absorption by the body. The higher the number—that is the glycemic index—the shorter the time taken for the conversion of the carbohydrate or sugars in the food to glucose for absorption by the body. If the glycemic index is low, the indication is that the body takes longer for the sugar content in that food to be absorbed. Glycemic index could therefore mean two things—one, the extent of carbohydrate or sugar content in a food, and two, the time taken by the body for release of the sugar content in it.

If there is no sugar content in a substance, the glycemic index of that is zero with water as an example of that. If the substance is plain concentrated sugar, then the glycemic index of that would be 100. All other foods are rated on a scale of one to hundred which implies that their glycemic index lies somewhere between that of sugar and water. There are some reports which indicate that some items do have glycemic index in excess of 100 like certain alcoholic drinks which are incidentally bitter tasting. Whether this is true or not, one thing is certain and it is that generally speaking the way a food tastes has nothing to do with its glycemic index. That is to say, simply because the glycemic index of a food is high does not necessarily mean it is sweet. Conversely, just because a food item is not sweet it does not follow that its glycemic index is low. Again there are sweetness-neutral foods with widely varying glycemic indices.

Among the food generally consumed, rice has a glycemic index of of around 70—say 60 to 80—depending on the variety of rice one uses with a particular type of rice referred to as Diabetic Rice having a much lower index. Wheat has an index of about 60 with the sugar content being almost the same as that of rice. This simply implies that wheat releases the sugar in it much slower than rice. This is the point to be taken note of. Since the glycemic index of wheat is lower than that of rice, we see rice eaters often being persuaded to shift to wheat in an effort to exercise greater control over their blood sugar levels. This is done so because lower glycemic index ensures longer time for absorption of the sugar in it by the body thus giving more time for the body's insulin to complete its work. Again as a strategy being put in place this change from rice to wheat will be beneficial since shifting to a food one is not used to will result in lower overall consumption thus aiding weight loss or at least avoiding weight gain. This we will see in detail later on.

As you would have guessed by now, vegetables particularly the leafy variety have all got low GI value in the range of 20 or so thus making them all fit candidates for consumption by diabetics. Cereals and pulses also have low GI values compared to rice with certain varieties of peas like Bengal Chana having a GI value of less than 10. From the angle of absorption of sugar by the body, one can see that these are splendid choices in the management of diabetes.

But the picture presented is not all that unidimensional with food to be taken only on the basis of glycemic index. Our body needs carbohydrates, fats, proteins, vitamins and minerals etc. for its proper functioning. One's settling for a diet plan should ensure that all the requirements are properly taken care of. Fat per se is not to be avoided. Fat gets accumulated over a period of time from out of the excess eating one indulges in from time to time. The point to be noted here is that carbohydrates are to be taken in on the basis of their GI value with low GI food preferred to high GI foods. That will be beneficial in the context of managing diabetes better. Carbohydrate starving as some people practice is to be avoided.

While discussing food, one should be aware of the fact that food items with the same GI value affects different persons differently. In order to complicate matters further, the same food has drastically different impact on metabolism when consumed in a different manner. Confused? No need to get puzzled. It is not all that complicated as we shall proceed to see now. The way a food item on its consumption affects the blood sugar level can be referred to as the glycemic impact.

Food items with a given GI value do exhibit varying glycemic impact depending on how it is consumed. While consuming some thing in its raw form will have low glycemic impact compared to it being taken in say a fried form, certain food items really show anomalous behaviour as far as its glycemic impact is concerned. As a case in point, let us proceed to examine how the glycemic impact of the same food item changes with the way it evolves in the process of its reaching your dining table. One ideal instance would be that of a variety of banana frequently used as part of one's every day diet in parts of South India. The banana in its raw form is used for making banana chips by deep frying it in oil and is also extensively used in the preparation of very many side dishes accompanying lunch. In its raw form it is classical green with its outer skin a shining green all over. It is often taken in boiled form accompanied by a little sauce or some thing like that. That is taking the raw banana boiled as it is. This is seen to have a beneficial impact on blood sugar levels of diabetics with tangible reduction in blood glucose levels almost always being brought about. In fact eating boiled raw banana is observed even to bring about hypoglycemia—a condition when blood sugar levels fall to alarmingly low levels—once in a while.

By way of a general phenomenon here it may be noted that blood glucose levels in a person registers its lowest level in 24 hours at around 3 a.m. Likewise, generally left to itself, it falls to its lowest level during day time by around 3 p.m. This will vary in the case of persons undertaking therapy for diabetes, though. The point here is one should be careful about taking food items like boiled raw banana in the evenings for fear of it aiding development of hypoglycemic conditions.

Back to banana, the very same banana which helps bring down blood sugar level when consumed raw makes your blood sugar levels to go up when consumed in its ripe form. On ripening the colour of its skin changes to bright yellow. The GI of ripe banana thus is much higher than its GI while it was raw. Again the GI of the ripe banana is found to increase steeply when it is consumed in its boiled form (This is a favourite diet of many in certain parts of South India and is an integral part of their breakfast) with one's blood sugar level really spiking and almost going through the roof. Given this situation, if somebody asks you if banana can be taken by a diabetic, it is difficult to give a one word answer for it.

The point to be noted is that the impact of food on metabolism depends on the manner in which it is taken—raw, ripe, boiled, fried, dry or in fermented form etc. By the way fermented foods generally show substantial hike in their GI value compared to its unfermented form.

Again, the impact of a food on blood sugar varies from individual to individual. For example, in a majority of cases sweet potato is seen to have beneficial impact on diabetics. But the minority is always seen to register much increase in blood sugar levels on consuming sweet potato. Taste is not a relevant factor as you would have seen by now—sweet potato reducing blood sugar and alcoholic drinks with bitter taste spiking blood sugar levels. Likewise most of the food items mentioned as being good or bad in general simplified suggestions to diabetics in matters of food choice are observed to have amazingly divergent effects from person to person. The only way to be sure of an item's impact on one's blood sugar is to monitor one's blood glucose level before and after consuming that food item on different occasions. This is comparatively easy these days with handy meters for checking of blood sugar with such meters easily available almost all over the place. The price of the testing strips are also poised for a steep fall in the near future.

6 MORE ON BLOOD SUGAR

T2D is the most prevalent form of diabetes with almost 95 per cent of diabetes falling under that category. T2D is a condition that develops over a period of time and it is almost always present in a person before it is formally diagnosed. In fact most people become aware of it while carrying out a general routine blood test done in the context of some other complaint reported for medical attention. The condition is given rise to by the decline in the efficiency of the beta cells of the pancreas in secreting insulin more often in conjunction with decreased insulin carrying efficiency of the carrier cells brought about by obesity among other things. As time goes by, the beta cells gradually begin secreting less and less insulin with the result that over a period time T2D is likely to catch up with every one. It is mentioned in a light vein that in case our longevity goes up to say a hundred and twenty years or so, the probability of every one getting T2D is close to hundred per cent!

T2D arises out of acquired propensity to get it to an extent, and the of life style followed by a person to a larger extent. Part of the former which can be labeled as the inheritance theory, I am sure that all of us would have heard quite a lot about. One's chances of getting T2D in case his or her parents or one of the great grandfathers were diabetics is what it is all about. While this is true to an extent, this is a bit far fetched also since ordinarily the great grandfathers would have passed off without any knowledge of their having diabetes because of diagnostic interventions being low in the past that far and also because of longevity issues associated with that period of time. This is not to question the validity of the heredity factor but to indicate that one need not be too much obsessed with that. Again, certain races are correctly held to be genetically predisposed to getting T2D. Like the Indians for example. While these are true one should admit that there is nothing much one can do about it. You have no choice over your parents and no choice of your race or country of birth. In that sense these are what one might call risk factors that can not be modified. Again with advancing age, as pointed out earlier the insulin secreting efficiency of the pancreas declines and this is another risk factor you have to live with even though its impact can be blunted by taking insulin shots. These are a given and nothing can be done about it. Or these are the non-modifiable risk factors.

What then are the modifiable risk factors? There are quite a few. These include your body weight, your eating habits and diet, the level of physical activity and most importantly your diabetic literacy and ability to undertake self-management. The importance of diet and exercise in the management of T2D has been often articulated by one and all. Again on the medicines front also, the importance of appropriate medication is also very well documented and practiced. T2D is to be seen and, understood and taken care of as a metabolic disorder which it certainly is. Like with all body functions, metabolism is a very complex activity at best only partially and peripherally understood. Factors known to medical science and very many factors yet to be unraveled affects the process called metabolism and this needs to be clearly understood. All the above factors mentioned as modifiable and unmodifiable risk factors affect your metabolism.

What is metabolism? Metabolism in a manner of speaking can be described as the process of converting our food intake into energy usable by our body. Simply put it is conversion of mass into energy using the processing capability of our digestive apparatus. The process is akin to the working of a nuclear reactor. You and I know what nuclear reactors are supposed to be doing. They convert an engineered loss of mass into its equivalent energy in a controlled environment generating some waste in the process. Well in a way this is what you and I have been doing continuously for very many years now.

The precautionary steps associated with a nuclear plant all of us are broadly aware of. At least we know that the activities associated with protecting this process of conversion of matter into energy is very complex and ensured to be error-free at huge cost. But what about the mini nuclear reactor you and I carry within each one of us? The complex functionality continues to perform marvelously despite all the abuse we subject our body to consciously or unconsciously. Poor little nuclear plant in each one of us is functioning with unflinching loyalty to us without the slightest hint of refusing to do its work.

The metabolic disorder—which is what diabetes essentially is—is influenced by very many activities which we engage in on a daily basis. To mention some of this would help clear things a little better. Regularity of habit is a factor which ensures smooth carrying out of metabolism to an extent. Eating at regular times helps immensely in streamlining the process, for example. Sleeping late at night—occasionally as well as on a continuous basis—results in blood sugar levels spiking unnecessarily and staying that way for long. Eating stale food is a major cause of metabolic dysfunction. Again, getting worked up and stressed out creates havoc in the metabolic activity.

These are but a few of the factors adversely affecting our metabolism. The interesting part of the story is that all these parameters are well within the realm of our total control. What is it that prevents us from eating at specific times every day? If there are issues associated with availability of food and such operational issues, identifying and addressing them should be taken up. Carrying food with you wherever you go is an option, for example. Eating stale food is in fact a matter of choice. Decide against eating stale food once and for all. Start doing it right now at your home if you are doing it and never ever go to eateries suspected of dishing out stale food. These are small little things within your control. These when done effectively and meticulously will do a lot of good for your general health as well.

Again, sleeping for about seven to eight hours a day is just a matter of choice and practice. Do away with the practice of keeping late hours. Make it a habit to go to bed reasonably early at say 10 p.m. or so at the latest and get up by about 5 a.m. or thereabout. Enjoy a siesta in the afternoon for about fifteen or thirty minutes if possible. Try to squeeze this into your routine. What you are now engaged in after 10 p.m. can be attended to in the morning since you can start your day early and afresh everyday. Attend to them the first thing on getting up. In fact your effectiveness in doing work earlier on in the day will be many times more productive compared to working late into the night.

As for stressing out, you can ensure that you set for yourself only realistic and reasonable targets capable of being achieved in the normal course. In matters personal, professional or related to work, do ensure that you do not bite more than what you can chew. Do not settle for deadlines that will add to your tension. For example, do not leave to catch a flight from an airport a half-hour way at the last minute. Plan your trips in such a way that you will reach your destination well within the required time without any hassles. In places where you have to be, make sure you have arrangements in place to ensure that you are there ahead of time. This will help you avoid build up of tension and make you relaxed as well. This may sound difficult, but in practice you will find that this is in fact very easy once you apply yourself properly to it. Tension builds up and you become stressed out largely on account of inept and inadequate planning, and from the health angle it will do you a world of good to plan for events without it adding unnecessarily to your tension.

Again for relieving stress, physical activity will come in very handy. Apart from bringing down your blood sugar levels by burning sugar directly, exercise of all kinds will help you reduce stress. It tones up your systems and equips you to take on your tasks at hand with confidence and reassurance. Stay focused on engaging in physical activities whenever and wherever possible even finding opportunities in the performance of small routine day-to-day activities. Using stairs instead of lift at least for traveling down in the office building, walking the steps while being in the shopping mall escalator are all small changes that add up to benefit you substantially. Parking your car a little away from where you have to get down helps you engage in walking a little distance. At home rather than calling your spouse and children to bring something or climbing the stairs to get something you need, cultivate the habit of doing it yourself. All these eventually add up to living in a more healthy way. It helps you a great deal in keeping yourself fit, energetic and more tuned to achieving success all around.

Then there is meditation to be taken up in right earnest. This is perhaps the greatest stress reliever of all. It helps your body maintain itself in an optimally functional manner. Meditation broken down to its element simply means putting your whole being—your heart and soul and whatever—into whatever you are doing at the present. It need not be performed in an isolated place or a place of worship or any thing like that. It can be done here and now but with full focus on it. Not an iota of your attention be allowed to go away from what you are doing now. You will then lose track of the flow of time with time appearing to be non-existent. Now as you are reading this book, if you are hundred per cent into it, this is meditation.

In the management of T2D, the requirement is medication and meditation and not medication versus meditation. In fact medication can be progressively brought down and meditation progressively stepped up. Meditation will get automatically stepped up whereas medication needs to be deliberately brought down.

7 T2D IS IT A DISEASE?

What is a disease? Disease literally means dis-ease, that is lack of ease. But over the years because of usage this has started taking the meaning of illness. Any condition that interferes with your ease is a disease. In fact people could be having some illness or other without it really interfering with one's ease in any manner. As a matter of fact we notice an illness only when it lowers your ease in carrying on the normal routine. In that regard the usage of disease as a synonym for illness is in order. May be that is how disease has got associated with illness. However our job is not to get involved with the etymology of disease. May be our question needs to be remodeled as "is T2D an illness?"

Let me answer first question first. T2D is not a disease simply because it seldom does interfere with your ease in the initial stages—in fact initial years—of its development. As pointed out earlier, a vast majority of the persons who have developed it are as yet unaware that they are having this condition. Remember very many who know that they have T2D came to know about it through routine blood tests conducted in connection with some health condition warranting that test? That is the way it is. It does not at all affect your ease ordinarily for a long long time. It's almost like asking is ageing a disease? It is in the sense that it interferes with your ease at some point of time late in life. But for that matter do you and I term ageing as a disease or illness?

Back to the questions at hand. Is Diabetes a disease or an illness? The answer is NO. It is not an illness in the sense that hunger is not an illness. It is not a disease in the sense that ordinarily for a very long while it does not interfere with your ease in carrying out your normal routine. If it is not a disease or illness, then what is diabetes? I would think rather than any thing else it is a metabolic disorder in much the same way as hunger. Only thing when you are hungry there is a metabolic disruption of order clamouring for an immediate solution. If not other forms of diabetes, at least T2D which constitutes about ninety five per cent of diabetes is a metabolic disorder and nothing more than that. It is a metabolic disorder that can be corrected in the same way as food intake takes care of hunger for a while. In the same manner we can have T2D corrected for a while by going in for appropriate changes in our habits. Like feeding your hunger at regular intervals, correct your T2D at regular intervals and the condition will not bother you at all.

The point here to be noted is that every body is looking out for cure for diabetes thinking it as an illness. If you have fever or say typhoid or pain in the foot or whatever, you have a cure for those conditions and looking out for a cure as such is in order. But

T2D is not a disease or illness in that sense. It is brought about by a combination of two aspects—the impairment of insulin secretion and the development of insulin resistance. Both these combine to result in a condition whereby the body is apparently deprived of the required levels of energy and blood deposited with increasing amounts of glucose.

So how do we tackle it? Obviously by improving the insulin secretion within the body, or by providing insulin from external sources to compensate the internal deficiency. Then we have to tackle whatever factors are contributing to insulin resistance and ensure that this is got out of from our path, right? Thirdly, we have to shake off whatever excess glucose is getting into the blood stream. For none of these there are magic cures. We have to manage our life style in such a way that these needs are addressed on a continuous basis so that we are free from the condition called T2D. As of now, there are no oral insulin available which shuts out the possibility of consuming it in the form of tablets. Only dependable source of external insulin is in the form of injections to be taken. There are some developments in the case of insulin sprays that can be inhaled, but they are in the testing stage and usability of that if and when available is expected to run into problems related to doze fixation so much so that it is also not a viable option. In any case matters related to insulin we will separately discuss. To start with we will consider what is it that we can do by way of activities within our control to improve insulin secretion and reduce insulin resistance.

It is a widely recognized fact that food correctly taken dispenses with the requirement of medical supplements in the ordinary maintenance of our body. This is quite true in the case of conditions that leads one to diabetes and also plays a significant role in the management of diabetes once you develop it. As you would already know, for managing obesity and to ensure that one's body weight is within permissible limits, we will have to look at a combination of two aspects related to life style. T2D is more of a lifestyle condition brought about by following a lifestyle unfriendly to the proper functioning of our bodily systems. First and foremost among the faulty aspects of our present day life style relates to the habits we follow in relation to food. This is actually three pronged. First of all it has to do with the nature of food we consume. Second it concerns with the frequency and quantity of the food we eat. Third it has to address the specific nutritious requirement of the body. We will take up one by one in detail and examine what would be the ideal recommended nature of these aspects.

8 THE FOOD WE TAKE

Diabetic or no diabetic, each of us has got certain perceptions about the food we take or at least supposed to take. For example, all of us somehow believe that sugar and thus carbohydrates should not be taken in excess. Likewise with salt also. Just about every one believes that it should not be consumed without limit. So on and so forth all of us have notions—right or wrong—about the kind of food that is good for our body. Not that we practice it always, but still we know that deviations in eating not in line with our belief are not good for us. Not only sugar and salt, in fact, every thing including not only food but every thing should be practised in moderation without having too much or too little for our comfort. But how far our notions are correct or validated with regard to the kind of foods we believe are to be avoided or consumed? Answering this question correctly may throw up a few surprises. Now let us proceed to examine each of the major categories of food we normally consume in a little detail.

Carbohydrate—Is it the villain?

The root cause of diabetes is that glucose supplied to us through the food we eat in the form of various sugars and carbohydrates somehow gets into the blood without it nourishing the body cells and tissues as usable energy which is absolutely essential for the body to continue its normal ordinary functioning. Such infiltration of glucose into our blood stream causes the blood glucose levels to rise beyond the permissible levels bringing with it a whole lot of problems some of which are of a non-reversible nature. This in a nutshell is what diabetes is all about. The problem here will appear on the face of it as carbohydrate intake. In case carbohydrate is not consumed as is being consumed now, probably there will not be enough glucose in the first place to get converted into sugar. In fact then there is no case or reason for blood sugar levels to rise beyond agreeable levels. This might appear to be correct but it really is far removed from truth. If one thinks of carbohydrate as the villain of the piece, then may be this argument holds good. Unfortunately a lot many people who have developed diabetes and are aware of their having developed it hold this view. For them less of carbohydrate means liberation from diabetes. Nothing is as far removed from truth as this.

To put matters in perspective, let us answer a simple question—is low carbohydrate intake associated with healthy living? The straight answer to the question is a firm NO. Carbohydrate is single handedly responsible for providing our body with all forms of energy for its normal healthy functioning. If our body can be considered as an engine—which it is not, this assumption is being made only to make things clear by an analogy—then carbohydrate is the fuel that runs it. Without carbohydrate the engine will cease to function like a motor car not fed with gasoline. Carbohydrate does function very many important and critical tasks in the functioning of the body and among them the most important function is that it maintains the functioning of our brain. Brain function goes completely haywire in case it is deprived of continuous supply of glucose. And that could be the reason why carbohydrates are found in everything we eat right from vegetables of all kinds to grains, pulses, milk and just about every thing except perhaps water, fish and meat.

Ranking on a par with oxygen and water, carbohydrates or glucose to be precise is absolutely essential for our survival. Glucose provides energy at the cellular level and without this our cellular functioning gets seriously impaired. How much of carbohydrates are necessary depends our energy requirement. The energy required consists of the energy required for maintenance of our base level bodily functions and the energy we need for the performance of activities outside our body which amounts to the energy required for the conscious acts being engaged in by us. This includes the performance of all work we engage in like walking, talking, eating and all types of movements. Our carbohydrate intake should be just about sufficient to take care of this. Any thing in excess of this will get stored as fat adding to body weight and it is not recommended. Any thing short of this will make you fatigued and fagged out. So the amount of carbohydrates you have to consume is dependent on your specific energy requirement. This we will have an idea of once you pay a little attention to your activities.

Arriving at the actual requirement of energy is only one part of the required information. The second part is the way you spend your energy. While the base level requirement of the body follows a general well known pattern, your activity level requirement of carbohydrate needs to be found out. Whatever the nature of the requirement, you can not just take in all the carbohydrate requirement in one shot. This is so because of two reasons. One, in case of just one shot your metabolic system will find it difficult to cope with the task of converting the carbohydrate into usable energy. This will require of the pancreas to have the full required quota of insulin to be made available in one shot and the released glucose carried to its destinations within the body in one go. Simply, this is an impossible task even in the healthiest of individuals. Second, your energy requirement is spread out in nature with the need for energy in a day unevenly spread over twenty four hours. For these two reasons your energy availability and hence carbohydrate infusion should be spread out over the day in tune with the body's changing requirements at various points of time in the day.

How this is achieved we will see in detail while discussing the concept of glycemic index and glycemic load while taking up recommended diet plan later on.

Fat isn't all that fatty

Fat again is a much maligned entity. Like we mentioned about carbohydrates, fat is also absolutely essential for the proper maintenance of our bodily functions. Without fat our systems break down and we will not be able to carry on living. The problem with the general aversion for fat is plain and simple lack of proper understanding of its various functions. One thing you can rest assured is that fat is very critical in the maintenance of health. Given the nature of discussions we are having here, we are not getting into the details of why it is important. But be informed that it is very very important.

From the angle of metabolism, conversion of food into fat takes place when the energy released from out of the food consumed is not spent as energy directly. Spending energy directly simply implies spending it for our base level requirements to carry out the ordinary body processes PLUS energy spent for external work carried out by us. To understand this better, let it be explained by drawing a comparison in financial terms. Think of the energy released from the food we consume as our income and energy consumed by the body as our expenses. The energy consumed is the total of energy required for the automatic bodily functions as well as the external work being done by the body. Suppose our income is more than our expenses, we end up with a surplus. Likewise if food is treated as energy in and work done as energy out, if work done is less than the energy coming in you end up with a surplus in energy. This surplus energy is saved. The only way it can be saved is as fat. You save your money by putting it in your safe, bank or in investments. Likewise the energy saved is stored as fat in various parts of the body—in your stomach area as paunch and other parts as flab.

Continuously having such excesses will transform to you gaining in body weight. Fat tends to accumulate and this accumulation has been resorted to by the body for very sound historical reasons.

Even though going into the reasons why fat is getting stored as it is is beyond the scope of this narration, we will have a brief look at it to put things in perspective. Body engages in conversion of surplus energy into fat for very sound reasons as we shall briefly see now. Fat is important for the only reason that close to two-thirds of our brain is made of fat. In India, it is almost ritualistic to have intake of ghee as part of one's regular food one way or the other. The fact that fat is the main content of the brain is the reason why generally Ayurvedic preparations targeting improvement in brain function of one kind or other is always administered in fatty form to ensure proper absorption. Fat is what helps us cope with prolonged stress—both physical and mental—and it also navigates us through periods of sickness, and deprivation of food intake. The storing mechanism, it is understood, has been resorted to by the body to see that life did not lose steam when confronted with starvation and deprivation of energy. During periods of famine and illness during the long evolutionary processes the human race has been through, fat is what held charge of navigating us through it all and held charge successfully. Otherwise I would not have been here to write this and you to read this. There are different kinds of fats and also healthy fats among them the consumption of which is actually recommended. This we shall see in detail later on.

9 WHAT TO EAT

Most people with diabetes are generally obese and over weight to start with. At a certain stage of the progression of the condition, owing to a combination of factors diabetics tend to look emaciated with a look of having completely depleted their energy almost all the time. But the major factor in a person becoming a diabetic in the first place is his being over weight and obese. Because of this, to prevent the onset of diabetes management and maintenance of body weight within permissible limits is of paramount importance. This is required not just to prevent the onset of diabetes but is the main factor around which management and eventual reversal of diabetes is to be brought about. Battling diabetes in a manner of speaking is in fact centered around systematic weight loss or weight reduction to start with. Weight reduction incidentally will bring about with it other benefits like reduced blood pressure, increased feeling of being energetic— because you have less weight to carry around !— improved mobility and even improved life expectancy. Central obesity or what is being referred to as Syndrome

X and metabolic syndrome is what is opening the gateway to most life threatening illnesses and also certain unhealthy conditions including diabetes.

While undertaking the journey down the weight reduction lane, one common problem that is encountered is the understanding about what constitutes normal weight. While there are ever so many technical tools like BMR, Body Mass Index (BMI) etc. associated with this, let us not get caught in all these. Instead let us start the weight loss programme here and now. Let us register progress in the direction of losing body weight in small quantities. Let us not aim at reducing weight by five kilos in the first month or so. Let us begin our task without caring for how much we are losing. For your information weight lost fast is also regained equally fast or even faster. So let us stick to our weight loss programme aiming for small weight loss but importantly on a sustainable basis. Your weight will be normal when your physical parameters will be normal as required by clinical tests. Let us work towards achieving normalcy all around—not just with regard to weight alone. You have normal weight when you will be truly energetic to take on the world in a spirit of enjoyment. When you feel laid back, lazy and have difficulty in coping with normal demands made on you, you can safely presume that you have a problem related to body weight—or simply your body weight is not normal. When things are not that way, your body weight is normal. No two individuals have the same physical characteristics and what is normal weight for me will not be normal weight for you. The concept of

BMR, BMI etc. are certain broad indicators to serve as our guide only.

We have seen that carbohydrates, fats, proteins, vitamins and minerals are absolutely essential for carrying out our normal bodily functions for our healthy living. There is a very popular and prevalent view among diabetics and people associated with the management of diabetes that carbohydrate intake is to be minimized if not avoided for taming diabetes. This view is very wrong. Roughly about fifty to sixty per cent of our food intake should provide us with carbohydrates. We have also seen that perhaps with the exception of water just about every thing we consume has got some carbohydrate in it. That is to say almost all food items we take contain ingredients of sugar in it. Our overall intake of all food materials should be giving us adequate carbohydrate to be converted into sugar for use by the body.

Suppose we take all the carbohydrate required by the body in one shot as plain sugar all at once, the result as you know would be spiking of our blood glucose levels. This is so because our body finds it difficult to handle this much of carbohydrate all at once and whatever is not made use of gets shifted to blood adding to the blood glucose level. Obviously this is not a very happy situation. This kind of situation is to be avoided in the interest of maintaining proper health. So what is it that needs to be done? We should give our body carbohydrates in quantities it can effectively make use of without adding to our blood glucose levels improperly. The quantities being fed should be more or less in tune with the level at which our body can make use of it for its energy requirement. That is to say the process of giving carbohydrate should be gradual and continuous and sustained all through the day everyday. How is this done? We will see it now.

We know that the glucose in sugar is absorbed very fast within minutes by the body. Glucose is the form of sugar that the body needs as fuel for conversion into energy. Any other form of sugar is consumed by the body only after it is converted into glucose. Then, what about the sugar in say rice or wheat? Or for that matter in potatoes or vegetables? You know that rice and wheat are not all sugar. They contain other ingredients as well. So is the case with potatoes and vegetables. If we consume rice or wheat or potatoes or vegetables, our body receives much less sugar compared to the situation where we would have taken an equal amount of plain and simple sugar. Again apart from the quantity of sugar released there is some delay involved in rice, wheat, potatoes or vegetables releasing as glucose the sugar contained in them. This is so because the sugar in these is not stored as glucose and our body has to first convert the sugar contained in these to glucose before it is ready for absorption by it for its functioning. Thus you can see that consuming rice or wheat or potatoes or vegetables results in one, less release of glucose for the body since they contain much less sugar compared to sugar itself and two, a longer time for release of glucose in it for absorption by the body because of the need to get the carbohydrates in that get converted into glucose.

Food items vary one another in terms of these two properties—one, the amount of carbohydrates present in it, and two, the time it takes for the carbohydrate in it to get converted into glucose. Simple carbohydrates get converted into glucose without delay whereas complex carbohydrates take time to get converted into glucose depending on their chemical structure. The less the quantity of simple carbohydrates you consume at any point of time the better for the body to assimilate it. Also, if the release of sugar by the carbohydrate takes longer and is extended in time the better equipped the body is to handle that without it in any way resulting in spiking of blood sugar level. Thus we can see that the impact a food has on the body in terms of influence on the blood glucose level is dependent directly not only on the level of carbohydrate contained in it but the nature of the carbohydrate also in relation to the time it takes for conversion into glucose for absorption by the body.

Glycemic Index or GI

Glycemic Index is a number given to a food item broadly indicating its impact on the blood sugar levels on consuming it. It can thus be taken as an indicator of the glycemic impact of a food item. Glycemic impact refers to the effect a food item has on increasing blood sugar level. On the basis of the carbohydrate content in a food material and the time taken by that content to get converted into glucose for absorption by the body, food items are classified by giving a number which broadly indicates these two aspects of a given food item. This is what is referred to as Glycemic Index or simply GI. Food items are classified in relation to sugar with sugar being given an index of 100. Other food items are given GI numbers depending on how much carbohydrate they contain and how fast that content gets converted into glucose in relation to plain sugar. In other words, it is an indication of how much carbohydrate a food contains and how fast it gets absorbed by the body. Accordingly rice is given a GI of around 70 and wheat slightly lower than that. Potatoes come in with an index of around 50 to 60 while leafy vegetables come in the range of 10 or so. These are only approximate indicators of how a food item affects the body by way of providing glucose to it. There is no hard and fast rules for this classification with these arrived at through observation of the effects of various food items on various persons. The GI value of different types of a given item also will vary significantly. Thus various varieties of rice will have varying GI with a variety mentioned in some places like Diabetic rice having a GI of less than 25. Again raw rice and unpolished rice have widely varying glycemic impact and hence varying GI. So also wheat as whole wheat powder called *rava* has a lower GI than wheat as fine powder referred to as maida. Again, how one uses a food item also brings about a change in GI. A classic example of this would be the case of raw banana with a GI of about 20 in the raw form reaching a GI of about 60 while it is ripe when it is taken as a fruit. Further when the same ripe banana is boiled and consumed—a favourite item in many parts of South India as part of breakfast—the glycemic impact shoots up with GI well beyond 80! The point to be understood here is that GI only gives a broad indication of how one's metabolism is likely to respond to the intake of a particular food item in relation to its behavior specific to blood glucose levels.

Glycemic Index can be considered as a broad indicator of how high a food raises blood glucose levels once it is consumed. High GI foods will cause blood glucose to rise shortly after they are consumed. However in healthy individuals these foods trigger insulin secretion and this results in the glucose being released getting converted into energy for use by the body. In such a case the blood sugar levels are maintained in the normal range only. But unless this energy is utilized for performance of work by the body, the energy ultimately gets stored as fat in the body. Either way this is considered undesirable. Build up of fat results in body weight and over a period of time this leads to what is referred to as insulin resistance which triggers the onset of diabetes. So also consuming foods with high GI places unnecessary stress on the pancreas with the result that the pancreas will eventually lose its efficiency in secreting insulin in response to glucose being provided in the body. Both the possibilities are to be avoided in the interest of maintaining proper health. In the case of one with diabetes consumption of high GI foods will straightway result in spiking of blood sugar level thus worsening the condition further. In all cases, we can therefore see that, going in for low GI food is considered eminently desirable. Low GI foods do not put any stressful demands on the pancreas and as a rule do not result in fat accumulation resulting from excessive glucose intake. More important, consumption of low GI foods aids significantly in the effective management of Type II Diabetes.

More on GI and food

The food we generally eat comprise carbohydrates, proteins and fat along with water, fibre and some minerals. Sugar is almost entirely carbohydrate and oils comprise almost all fats. But, in general, the food we consume contain two or more of these ingredients. Carbohydrates, fats, proteins and minerals all impact one's blood glucose levels but their impact vary significantly. While plain and simple sugar almost immediately impact blood glucose level, other complex carbohydrates take up to an hour or more to impact depending on the nature of the carbohydrate present. Fat in contrast takes about three hours to have any noticeable impact on blood glucose level. Fat and proteins impact blood glucose much less significantly but they impact all the same. The Glycemic Index of a given food depends on how much of carbohydrate, fat, fibre and protein are present in it and how complex that carbohydrate is. Fibre significantly slows down the motion of food within digestive apparatus and hence delays release of sugar from it. Thus foods rich in fibre will have correspondingly low GI value.

If so, in view of the very low level of sugar contained in them, can one consume fat and protein without any restriction? No even from the angle of maintaining blood glucose within permissible levels, it is not at all advised. In the name of consuming less sugar you can not and should not consume protein and fats by way of food indiscriminately. For one, in that case your food intake in terms of sugar will be very low and you will be depriving yourself of a vital ingredient required for proper maintenance of your body. You have to take every thing in a balanced way, in moderation that is. You can not and should not have an all-protein or an all-fat diet. Because in that case many of your body functions will get badly affected. In fact in nature nothing is available in its pure form and you never get pure carbohydrate, pure fat or pure protein. We process naturally available stuff into processed this and processed that. This in itself is not really good for health. The more a food item is processed, the more its capability to harm your body.

Diabetes being a metabolic disorder related to one's endocrine system, it is inextricably linked to carbohydrate, lipid and protein metabolism. A high fat diet is considered to be one of the main reasons for development of insulin resistance paving the way for early onset of diabetes. Indiscriminate eating habits coupled with sedentary living can be considered the most important causative factor for the onset of Type 2 Diabetes. As a self-management tool and as a strategy in overcoming Type 2 Diabetes, eating properly taking care to avoid excess eating and eating the right kind of food assumes an important and very significant role in the management of Type 2 Diabetes. Proper management of diet is in fact adequate to maintain blood glucose levels in the normal range and to avoid all associated complications of Type 2 Diabetes.

Coming to the food choices before a Type 2 Diabetic, the guiding principle should be to limit carbohydrate intake as far as possible to high-fibre, low-fat carbohydrates. A diet containing such carbohydrate can dramatically improve one's overall health and hold blood glucose level in check. Fibre or what is referred to as roughage has several health benefits. For one, they do not add any calories to your food. They help slow down the digestive process and thus slow down release of glucose into blood. Fibre also gives a feeling of fullness or satiation thus satisfying your hunger without much addition by way of calories. Examples of fibrous carbohydrates include all grains and oats. Unprocessed grains often do have more roughage and thus they should be preferred to processed grains. Almost all fruits and vegetables are rich in fibre and are thus advised for consumption in the management of Type 2 Diabetes. The longer it takes for a food item to release the sugar in it, the lower its glycemic index. Thus unprocessed grains and cereals and almost all fruits and vegetables rank far lower in glycemic index and are recommended for intake as part of the management of Type 2 Diabetes. Higher intake of fruits and vegetables and fibrous foods is associated with significantly improved glycemic control. Any eating programme factoring this in decreases the risk of developing Type 2 Diabetes in the first place and helps improve effective self-management in persons who already have Type 2 Diabetes.

Low glycemic index alone is not the only aspect to be taken care of. How much of a food one eats also is quite important. Suppose you are replacing one unit of food with glycemic index of say 80 with two units of food with glycemic index of say 50, in fact you are going to have an elevated blood glucose level that will be higher in comparison with the situation if you had taken only one unit of food with higher glycemic index. That is to say, how much you eat is as important as what you are eating. For a given amount of food or portion being consumed, it helps if the glycemic index of the food is lower. This is to be specially taken note of. The portion size is really important. Again, achieving weight reduction can have significantly high impact in the efficient management of Type 2 Diabetes. Since fat consumption is definitely resulting in weight gain, care should be taken to ensure that even in cases of glycemic index being low, the fat content in the food is not high. Otherwise the beneficial impact of low glycemic index food intake will be more than offset by the contrary overall impact of high fat food intake.

10 EATING CHOICES

This is a question generally asked by diabetics and even others who are wanting to shed body weight, improve lipid profile and so on. Let us make one thing very clear at this point—you can not have a prescription made categorically like you can take this, this and this but can not take or not dare look at this, this and this food item. You might be wondering what is the harm in saying that one affected by Type 2 Diabetes should not be taking sugar, for example. Well you must have noticed that individuals who have been in the grip of Type 2 Diabetes for long and who are administered insulin once in a while collapse because of sugar levels falling quite low with the need to feed them with sugar for their recovery. That is to say, you can not maintain that a Type 2 Diabetic should never be given sugar. Even apart from medical emergencies like hypoglycemia we discussed above when blood sugar levels fall to dangerously low levels, there is no case for completely prohibiting intake of any kind of food for any one. For one, placing restrictions like don't take this, don't take that etc. are often counter-productive with the natural tendency of people to fight such compulsive directives. For another, metabolism itself is not very clearly understood by science to have such blanket embargos being put in place without a proper understanding of the processes involved while consuming a food. Yet another very important aspect not to be lost sight of is that our body needs a wide variety of nutrients that any restrictions put in place should not affect our body functions adversely. Why say at length when we have to ensure that even a chronic diabetic needs to be given sugar-releasing food regularly in order to keep him alive and ticking.

The point to be noted here is that the way an individual responds to a food or a particular kind of food varies from person to person. Again, the same food has got different glycemic index and insulin index depending on the manner in which it is consumed. For example, banana eaten raw reduces the blood sugar levels in most people while when ripe or boiled, it results in steep increase in blood sugar levels in almost all individuals. Likewise whole grain bread increases blood glucose levels much more slowly compared to white bread. Given this kind of situations, how can one precisely and satisfactorily answer a question whether banana or bread is safe or desirable for consumption by diabetics?

Similar is the case with regard to fruits and food preparations making use of jaggery. There is a school of thought which maintains that consumption of fruits is fine since they do not ordinarily contain glucose in it in that form. It is also indicated that the carbohydrate in fruits gets transformed into glucose for absorption by the body only after some bodily processes involving some delay and therefore they can be safely consumed without much adverse effect on the blood sugar levels. Same is argued to be the case with jaggery added foods as well. This argument is valid in general. But that does not mean that one affected by Type 2 Diabetes can have a free go at all fruits indiscriminately. Fruits generally contain carbohydrates as fructose and this needs to be got converted into glucose for absorption by the body. This conversion of fructose into glucose takes place only after a little while after being inside our body. Hence the glycemic index of these fruits are less compared to foods releasing glucose directly. Still yellow fruits like mangoes, pineapple and jackfruit are to be taken with care. Not that they will result in spiking of blood sugar immediately on consumption but that one has to monitor their effect on one's blood sugar independently before taking a view in the matter. This is all the more so because, as already stated, different foods behave differently in the case of different persons and thus nothing can be stated as a general rule in the matter of food selection from the angle of their glycemic impact. While consuming yellow fruits elevates the blood sugar levels in a very large number of cases, it is seen that the elevation in levels is generally not very steep or alarmingly high. The point that needs to be emphasized here is how one's system responds to a food in terms of its effect on blood sugar levels needs to be explored and determined individually in respect of each person.

The impact of a food item on one's blood sugar level can be ascertained by checking one's blood sugar level before and after consuming it. While testing before eating the food item is easy and straight, testing the one after food is taken is to be carried out within 90 to 120 minutes after consuming the food item. The test is ideally carried out for two or three or even more occasions before one can legitimately conclude about the impact of a particular kind of food on one's blood glucose level. In this connection it should be very clearly understood that the same food can have different effects on the blood glucose levels of different persons and as such glycemic indices of food items are only taken as indicative guidance for one to choose one's food appropriate to his system. The actual impact of a food item on an individual should be arrived at by resorting to the test mentioned above.

While this is so, based on the most prevalent practices and published glycemic indices and insulin indices of common food items, certain broad guidelines can be worked out about what foods can generally be consumed to hold one's blood sugar level in the acceptable range. This is a very vital part of self-management of Type 2 Diabetes. We will proceed to examine this now. However the issue of how to consume these food items and more importantly how much to be consumed we will see in continuation to this.

Broadly speaking, glycemic index is indicative of how fast the carbohydrate in a food gets converted into glucose while inside the body. Foods that are digested slowly release the carbohydrate in them and hence glucose on conversion of that slowly into the body and are thus maintained as having low glycemic index. When a low glycemic index food is taken, it gives time for the pancreas to release insulin and thus the blood glucose level can be maintained in a normal range. Also if release of glucose is slow and in tune with the performance of muscular work the glucose even if released to the blood without intervention of insulin can get itself burnt out without creating any problems as far as blood sugar level is concerned. On the other hand, foods that are digested fast and which contain large amounts of carbohydrate release larger amount of glucose into the body and that too very fast. This type of foods place heavy demand on the pancreas by way of insulin requirement. Failure to release sufficient amount of insulin results in bulk of the glucose finding its way into the blood stream thus spiking the blood glucose levels and kick-starting problems all around. Consequently these food items have high glycemic indices.

Examples of low glycemic index foods include almost all leafy vegetables, peas, beans, green gram, black gram, horse gram, onion and most fruits. Rice, wheat and all grains and pulses have their glycemic index in the medium range. High glycemic index foods include all kinds of sugars, almost all pastry items and most roots including potatoes. The glycemic index of a food item increases when the carbohydrate content in it is rich in glucose. This is so because the glucose in that food gets absorbed by the body as it is—that is directly as given. The sweetness in most fruits is on account of not glucose but fructose and as such before absorption by the body that needs to get converted into glucose. This process of conversion takes time and this is not done all of a sudden. Thus the sweetness in fruits is released to the body in a consumable form over a period of time in slow doses. Because of this the impact of the sugar in fruits on spiking the blood glucose level is significantly low resulting in the glycemic index of almost all fruits being in the low to medium range even in cases where the fruits themselves are sweet in taste. However compared to other fruits the glycemic indices of yellow fruits like pineapple, mango, jackfruit etc. are found to be high compared to other fruits.

Apart from glycemic index what affects blood glucose level is the portion size of the food one takes. For example the impact of taking one slice of bread on blood sugar will be less than the impact of taking two slices of bread even though as far as glycemic index is concerned both have the same glycemic index. Thus the portion size is also very important in maintaining blood glucose under check. Glycemic index is important in the context of enabling one to switch over from high glycemic index foods to low glycemic index foods in the choice of foods only. The overall impact of one's food consumption on one's blood glucose level depends on the quantity of food consumed as well. For a given quantity of food intake, it helps to go in for low glycemic index foods because it gives a feeling of fullness or satiation without loading oneself with too much sugar or too many calories. This helps one keep a check on the overall glycemic load as well without feeling hungry or without having a feeling of deprivation.

The glycemic load—the overall impact by way of sugary intake—of a portion size of food can be reduced by adding low glycemic index food to the portions taken without actually reducing the portion size. Adding onion liberally in a dish with potatoes can be given as an example. This is one option. If this option is followed one will have a filled feeling without unduly adding to the glycemic load. The easiest way to achieve this is to add fibrous food to the food intake. Low glycemic index options like oats, unprocessed cereals etc. are very good options that can be tried out. The best option in this regard is to consume some flax seeds just ahead of one's regular meal. This would substantially jack up the time taken for digestion of the food consumed along with that and thus ensure that release of glucose to the system is stretched out. This alone is observed to facilitate maintenance of blood glucose level in an acceptable range in a majority of cases of persons under the grip of Type 2 Diabetes.

11 ON EATING, AGAIN

When addressing the question of what to eat, people often ask to provide a list of what not to eat. Avoiding primary sugar is very important and accordingly only for plain sugar as it is it is a strict NO-NO. Other than this all foods can be finding a place in a proper eating plan. One should remember that carbohydrate is essential for the normal functioning of the body and the human brain accepts only glucose as its fuel. So avoiding carbohydrate is not at all recommended even though some Type 2 Diabetics are practising it with avoidable harmful consequences. Again, at the emotional level one should not have a feeling of deprivation as this would stand in the way of having a proper eating plan in place and getting it stabilized. The magic formula to be observed in this context is to monitor and limit the serving size or portion size of carbohydrate rich food.

Exclusive protein foods and foods high in protein are to be only carefully factored into a proper eating plan for Type 2 Diabetics. All Type 2 Diabetics are at high risk for developing kidney complaints and excessive protein intake can make the job of kidneys unnecessarily taxing. Different food items impact differently with respect to their impact on one's blood sugar level. This is essentially on account of the composition in terms of carbohydrate, fat, protein etc. of various items of food and equally importantly the manner in which one's body responds to these ingredients. All in all, before deciding on a choice of food item suited to you, first of all your response in terms of effect on your blood glucose should be found out by measuring blood glucose levels before and after consuming it. However, by way of a general guideline, we can maintain that foods that contain large amounts of primary glucose—examples being sugar, candies, all kinds of sweets—, pizzas, almost all Chinese foods served in restaurants, all pastry and meat items all fried items, all kinds of high fat foods, all kinds of high protein foods, coffee and tea are considered as being better minimized if not entirely avoided. Again before taking a final call on any food item as to be totally avoided one should be very clear about its impact on one's blood sugar level and this is possible by simply measuring the blood glucose level before and after taking it. One can get a fairly good idea of the glycemic impact of a particular kind of food on one's blood glucose only that way. The available published data about glycemic index are at best only broadly indicative of the likely glycemic impact of various food items on a majority of individuals, and that is only to be treated as such and not as conclusive and final. Like mentioned earlier also, it should be very clearly borne in mind that each one reacts to a particular kind of food in a unique manner as far as its impact on blood sugar is concerned whatever be its whatever index. Fixing up an eating plan and finalizing the composition of food one should follow to hold one's blood sugar under control should factor in this point.

The glycemic impact of the foods mentioned above which are better minimized or avoided can be substantially lowered by adding flax seeds or other soluble fibre, oatmeal, green salad fruits and vegetables or nuts to them or consuming these ahead of their intake. Proper selection of nuts and vegetables will ensure that the nutritional balance is maintained in your diet as well. Then there are very often divergent views expressed about the consumption of tea, coffee and alcoholic beverages. As regards soft drinks are concerned there does not appear to be much of confusion since there is a broad assessment that consumption of soft drinks is not desirable in the context of any effort directed at maintaining blood glucose level within reasonable limits. Not only that, even from the stand-point of maintaining general health these drinks including their diet-varieties are rightly held to be better avoided. While there is near unanimity with regard to the undesirability of consuming soft drinks, that is unfortunately not the case with tea, coffee and alcoholic drinks. The unanimity here is only in respect of the agreement that consumption of tea, coffee or alcoholic drinks will not improve one's blood sugar control. For us that is not enough. So let us look at it a little closely.

While high glycemic index foods or fast carbs as they are sometimes called convert the carbohydrate in them into glucose rather quickly, low glycemic index foods or slow carbs generally gets almost fully utilized as energy without the carbohydrate content in them getting passed on to the blood as blood sugar or in its absence stored as fat. This is happening so because of the carbohydrate conversion into glucose being broadly in tune with the energy requirement of the body. When the fast carbs get converted into glucose, if they are not consumed as energy for the work performed by the body, the excess glucose gets converted into energy where the insulin is sufficient for such conversion and this energy when not utilized gets stored in the body as fat. When there is not sufficient insulin to handle the excess intake of carbohydrate, the glucose released is emptied into the blood stream thus spiking blood sugar level. But in this scheme of things, where do coffee, tea and alocohol fit in? Except for the sugar content that is present as lactose in coffee and tea (the variety with added milk), there is nothing much to warrant a high glycemic index stamping for coffee, tea or alcohol. An issue to be accounted for here is why black coffee or black tea or for that matter lemon tea or herbal tea are considered as displaying characteristics similar to food stuff having high glycemic index? These should be having low glycemic index going by sugar content in that. Same is the case with alcohol also. That is to say, these drinks should be treated as safe for consumption by Type 2 Diabetics. While a view can be conclusively taken on this only after a study of its impact on each individual, as a general rule, blood glucose levels are seen to go up considerably on consuming all kinds of tea, coffee and alcohol.

Some glycemic index data providers give a very high glycemic index rating for alcoholic drinks probably based on the impact alcoholic beverages have on individuals chosen for their observation and study. While this may have exceptions based on individual response to alcohol at times, it is recommended to avoid consumption of alcoholic drinks to have better control exercised over one's blood glucose level. Type 2 Diabetics are advised generally to be consciously moderate in their consumption of alcoholic drinks. While blood glucose level spike usually noticed after intake of alcoholic drinks is perhaps the result of attendant consumption of food going up and also such food consumption tending to be indiscriminate, one can safely maintain that consumption of alcohol in no way helps one to control blood glucose level in any manner. In fact the opposite of this—blood glucose level going up sharply on consumption of alcoholic beverages—is observed in very many cases. Hence it is recommended to avoid, and if that is not possible for whatever reason, to limit and minimize consumption of alcoholic drinks in any efficient self-management of Type 2 Diabetes.

Now, let us take a look at coffee and tea. As mentioned earlier, coffee and tea whatever the glycemic indices allotted to them, are found to significantly raise the blood glucose level in almost all cases of consumption by not just Type 2 Diabetics but by just about everyone. Coffee and tea even in their black versions are basically stimulants the stimulating effect essentially stemming from the caffeine content in it. It whips the body on to a state of alertness as some people put it, but this is brought about by triggering an increase in blood pressure, elevated heart beat and worst of all bringing about a spike in blood glucose level. The nutrient value of coffee, tea (and also alcohol) is nothing to write home about while the damage these items do to our body and its systems is immense. Stimulants add to the body's stress and thus adversely impact the metabolic process as a whole. While starting the day with a tea or coffee as practiced widely by a majority of people is obviously the wrong way to start a day, for a Type 2 Diabetic, starting a day like that is to be strictly avoided in case one hopes to manage his blood glucose level in a healthy manner. As mentioned coffee, tea and alcohol are addictive and it is difficult but not impossible to phase out the consumption of these over a period of time. For a Type 2 Diabetic his blood glucose control improves with the phasing out of tea and coffee in all cases without fail, and for this reason alone all Type 2 Diabetics should actually avoid tea and coffee in any form. This will go a long way in helping him maintain his blood glucose level within a permissible healthy range.

12 HOW TO EAT?

Eating starts at the point when our mouth gets in touch with what we are eating. Our mouth is not just a place to receive whatever we want to eat. It is not that the mouth is expected to pass on to the alimentary canal whatever it is fed with. It does pass on for sure. But its job is not simply to pass on whatever it receives as it is. Whatever is fed into the mouth is expected to be subjected to some value addition while inside the mouth and before being passed on to the digestive system for absorption by the body.

The basic requirement of any eating is that whatever is eaten is to be used by the body. Broadly speaking, food that is not properly used up by the body is the major contributor to fat build up and weight gain. If the food we eat is fully processed and utilized by our body, weight gain and by extension of that all problems attendant to that will not occur. To facilitate proper absorption and thereafter proper metabolism of carbohydrates in our food, we have to first ensure that the value addition expected to take place in the mouth does in fact take place. The value addition essentially comes from chewing the food properly for an interval of time. During this interval enzymes will get combined with the food thereby ensuring proper processing of the food inside our body. As far as carbohydrate is concerned, when we chew the food an enzyme in our saliva gets activated and the carbohydrate accompanied by this enzyme is readied for proper absorption by our body. In case if the food is not chewed properly or if it is simply slid down our throat without coming into contact with saliva as most people often do you have a problem on your hand. Whatever you eat that way—at least a significant portion of that in any case—gets eventually parked as fat somewhere in your body. Over a period of time this results in weight gain opening the flood gates of very many illnesses. Fat cells do remain in the body once they are given rise to and any reduction in fat achieved is brought about by not flushing out fat cells but by only shrinking it. So unnecessary build up of fat cells if not allowed to be formed in the first place, can help avoid a lot of problems down the line.

Foods can be eaten in raw, boiled and fried forms. Foods of plant origin—all vegetables and fruits—are better eaten in their raw form or closer to raw form. Our system has been accustomed to getting foods of plant origin in its raw form for thousands of years and consuming these items in the raw form is the best way to ensure that they are properly digested and the energy along with nutrients in them are properly absorbed by the body. Moreover, vegetables and fruits in their raw form contain very many enzymes which promote their easy absorption within our body. Boiling it or cooking it in any manner will cause diminishing the presence of and at times completely take away these enzymes thus making their proper absorption by the body incomplete, difficult and even impossible.

Foods of plant origin are advised to be taken in their raw form as far as possible. Even when they are boiled or otherwise cooked it is recommended to have them maintained near their raw form without heating or cooking them much. What is best avoided is frying since frying makes food lose its enzymes almost completely without a trace. Frying a food item therefore makes it difficult to get digested, and when digested with great difficulty after unnecessarily and mercilessly taxing our digestive system, they seldom have any positive impact on our body because of the heavy load of fat content in anything eaten fried. What is even more harmful is that whatever fats are used for frying also get spoilt while deep heating it and turn harmful after being inside our body. Again, a very widely prevalent habit of frying food items in oil which has been earlier used for frying is extremely harmful for one's body. This kind of eating of food items not only adds to undue weight gain but also incites the possibility of the onset of many debilitating deceases which are referred to as life-style deceases in which Type 2 Diabetes also finds a place. Other medical conditions in the group include lopsided lipid profile, elevated blood pressure, nephrological complaints and even cancer to name a few. The point is that fried foods of all types if avoided will do our health a world of good. Foods of animal origin are, like fried foods, better minimized if not avoided altogether in any efficient self-management of Type 2 Diabetes.

Summing up, do make it a point to eat slowly whether or not you are a Type 2 Diabetic. Eat slowly enjoying your food, chewing it well and appreciating the various qualities of the food while chewing it. Invoking the blessings of God and thanking him while beginning to eat one's food which was a part of the custom widely prevalent and practiced as a matter of religious requirement has been doing all a lot of good in at least with regard to our maintaining a healthy eating habit. Never ever eat in a hurry as that is the worst thing that can happen to the food and also to your digestive system. The body needs some time to register and communicate to you that its hunger is satiated. If you keep on hurriedly eating without giving this space for your body, whatever you eat in this interval goes on to get stored in your body as fat.

Another point to be noted here is that saliva tends to get reduced with advancing age. That is the contribution of enzymes from chewing will be progressively diminishing. To overcome this deficiency one has to chew one's food even more to ensure that the required enzymes are added to the extent required while sending the food inside. Unfortunately the onset of Type 2 Diabetes also synchronises with this advancing age which makes it even more important to have food properly chewed in particular with advancing age.

13 WHEN TO EAT?

Once you have decided what to eat and how to eat, the next important point is when to eat. We have seen that the matter is being discussed here as part of an effective way to manage Type 2 Diabetes. We have also seen that Type 2 Diabetes is a condition largely brought about by insulin resistance which in turn is contributed by a combination of one or more factors from among physical inactivity, overeating and obesity. All these three factors are instrumental in one putting on excessive weight which is often accompanied by what is called central obesity or Syndrome X or metabolic syndrome. Any serious attempt at tackling Type 2 Diabetes—also metabolic syndrome which is the forerunner of many debilitating physical conditions—should therefore address this issue. Naturally the focus of managing Type 2 Diabetes effectively is on bringing about sustainable weight reduction and getting out of the metabolic syndrome. While getting out of metabolic syndrome and its associate central obesity is to be largely addressed by resorting to appropriate physical exercises, weight loss is to be primarily addressed by changes to be brought about in eating habits. Having had a look at the what and how of eating, let us now look at when to eat so that sustainable weight loss is achieved.

While giving shape to a weight loss plan one has to be realistic. Attempting to lose weight fast is often unrealistic and harmful to the body. Again, weight that is lost fast is also likely to return fast. What we should be aiming at is sustainable weight loss. Losing weight to the extent of about a kilogram a fortnight or two kilograms a month will be an ideal target to start with. This can be set as the goal till such time one reaches a reasonable level of weight commensurate with one's height. BMI or Body Mass Index is an ideal reference that can be made in this regard by way of arriving at the reasonableness of one's body weight. It is a rather straight forward and simple way of working out what can be considered as one's reasonable weight. One's BMI is his weight in kilograms divided by his height in metres twice—that is to say weight in kilograms divided by height in metre squared. For example, if one's weight is 70 Kg. and height is six feet—that is 180 centimetres or 1.8 metres—the corresponding BMI is 70 divided by 1.8 once and again by 1.8. This equals 21.60. That is the corresponding BMI. This is a calculation you can do at the back of your hand or at least using your mobile phone quite easily. A BMI of up to 23 is considered ideal with a BMI above 27 considered clearly overweight. BMI in excess of 35 is what is referred to as obese.

Our body expects close to three-fourths of the energy consumed by it during day time. That is to say the body needs to be fed with food in such a manner that it is provided with about seventy five percent of its energy requirement from the moment you wake up till such time you go to bed. The requirement of energy is almost uniform during this period, and the requirement starts from the moment you get up. So one must start eating close to the time one gets up say within about thirty minutes or so. Does this amount to saying that one should start eating more since normally people begin to eat only quite some time after waking up? No, not at all.

We are starting to eat immediately on waking up to supply our body with the energy to take on the day. This is part of an overall strategy of spacing out eating without in any way increasing the overall quantity of food taken. What we are trying to do is to have our body supplied with food in a uniform manner all day long. Down the years we have somehow developed the habit of having three large meals a day—breakfast, lunch and dinner. What we are doing that way is to dump food into our system only thrice in a day against the actual requirement of food more or less uniformly spread over the entire day time.

One should therefore change the eating schedule by eating as many times a day as possible without however increasing the overall intake of food. Something like eating every two hours will ensure that you are supplying your system with food in tune with its requirement. Think of the situation our body is going through everyday day after day. We have seen that the requirement of energy is by and large spread over uniformly all through the day. Have you ever imagined how the body is coping with this at present? The question is specially relevant for Type 2 Diabetics. We are unloading food into our digestive system in bulk some time in the morning as breakfast. By noon we do the same thing and call it lunch. Come evening or night, the same thing is repeated and call it dinner. All this while your body is expending energy in much smaller quantities compared to the energy supplied by the food on all three occasions. What happens to the energy remaining unutilized at the point of eating? Your body has no other option but to convert it into fat and store it at some available part in the body. This results in fat mass which accumulates over a period of time taking you to a situation where you are likely to develop not just diabetes but very many other difficult conditions. If you can not have sufficient insulin in your body or the carrying capacity of cells carrying insulin is impaired in some way, you have a problem on your hands straightway on eating with bulk of the sugar in the food that you eat on the three occasions finding its way into your blood thus elevating your blood glucose to dangerous levels. Now, imagine your eating your food spread over as many times as possible—say during ten occasions uniformly spread over the day time. Your body will then be able to handle the food well by putting to optimum use the energy released. Importantly, it may be noted that the insulin demand on your body in such a situation also is limited. Even if some energy finds its way into your blood elevating your blood sugar level the work performed by your muscular mass for the routine activities will ensure that your blood glucose levels are not getting spiked. Thus you can see that it is eminently more scientific and sensible for every one to have food taken spread across as many times as possible and the beneficial effects by following that practice are enormous for a Type 2 Diabetic.

Spreading out one's eating over as many times as possible is highly effective in preventing formation of fat cells and fat mass and this helps keep weight under check on a sustainable basis. Again, this is a very important gain for a Type 2 Diabetic. However, care should be taken to ensure that the aggregate amount of food taken is never allowed to exceed the current level to start with. The infusion of whatever food you are taking as of now should be first spread over as many times as possible taking care to ensure that the overall amount of food taken is not exceeding the current consumption spread across the breakfast, lunch and dinner put together. This way you can preempt the formation of fresh fat and ensure that the food you eat is almost fully consumed by your body for utilization as energy. The bonus is that your digestive apparatus also will be thankful to you for not taxing it in a heartless manner with heavy loads of food in the morning, afternoon and evening. Now that you spread out your eating it can go about doing its job at a very leisurely pace. Your pancreas also will be much relieved in that demand made on it for insulin also will be minimal. Even though more the number of times you eat without adding to your overall intake of food is the best thing to do, taking into account the practical problems associated with that in a lifestyle you are used to this far, as a beginning effort should be made to ensure that you keep eating small portions of food every two hours. By this practice alone you will see that any tendency to put on weight is automatically reversed and over a period of time you start losing a kilogram or two every month without any extra effort. You will enjoy your new light feeling which is more than sufficient to keep you motivated in continuing with your new habit of eating frequently. For Type 2 Diabetics the gradual reduction in their blood sugar level will come as a great relief as well. This reduction is actually fully sustainable and brought about only through spacing of one's food and nothing else. Type 2 Diabetics will also like others find themselves having more energy at their disposal with their routine chores attended to with greater enthusiasm. While initially continuing with the eating composition as at present, gradually one can work out changes in the composition of food as mentioned in the previous chapter on what to eat. Type 2 Diabetics should gradually factor in the low glycemic index high soluble fibre foods into their food choices and would then be delighted to see their blood glucose levels being maintained very close to the normal permissible levels. No major changes need be brought in at this stage by eliminating foods that you love eating, but care should be taken not to overload your food composition with high glycemic index foods and foods that on one's testing have been found to result in spiking of blood sugar level. Over a period of a month or two a stable eating schedule should be firmly in place in terms of eating frequency as well as variety in content and taste at the same time ensuring low glycemic load. If this is followed, a Type 2 Diabetic would have achieved a measure of success in the self-management of diabetes on a sustainable basis. You should in all probability be on your way to managing your blood glucose levels effectively.

Spacing out eating by distributing whatever food consumed now—never attempt any reduction in the total quantity of food you take in a full day, to start with and do not try to change the component of foods you are used to again to start with—to as many times as possible is the first step in bringing about dietary changes aimed at effectively managing Type 2 Diabetes. The more the number of times the better and more uniform the availability of energy for carrying out our bodily functions. So also, this ensures that insulin requirement is reduced to the minimum apart from almost completely eliminating the possibility of fat build up and weight gain. This one step in itself will ensure substantial control being exercised in maintaining blood glucose within permissible levels. The fact that you are not disturbing or reducing your normal food intake in a day will ensure that you will not have any kind of feeling of deprivation normally associated with dietary changes. This will help you get into the new routine without any kind of reservation or apprehension. As a matter of fact frequent eating will make you think that you are indulging in eating a little too much and this often brings about the desired reduction in portion sizes automatically.

Now we will proceed to examine the number of times one should be taking food. As stated already, ideally it is best to maximize the number of times. However to put this in practice there are obvious problems associated with this. Hence as a first step one can start taking food six times a day in place of the three times most people are used to as of now. This should not be really difficult and people who have adopted this practice are seen to enjoy it and stick to it. This simple step facilitates weight reduction in not just the case of a Type 2 Diabetic but in just about all cases of persons practicing it. Even after doing this for a couple of days one tends to feel more energetic and would without any difficulty continue with this habit. After all you are being asked to eat more frequently and not to go without food! To that extent it is really a welcome proposition. But remember, the aggregate food intake in a day should not be increased. What you are eating spread over three occasions now should be spread over six occasions. That's all.

Now the next question arises—how to spread your eating into six occasions? At what time intervals one should be eating? Assuming that one sleeps for about eight hours a day, food consumption should ensure regular availability of adequate amounts of energy during the remaining sixteen hours in a day. In this time band one should commence eating within about half an hour of waking up and wind up eating for the day about two hours before going to bed at night. For example, if you get up at 6 a.m., you can have some light eating before 6.30 a.m. followed by your breakfast by about 8.30 a.m. There can be an in-between snacking by 10.30 a.m. followed by lunch around 12.30 noon. Some snacks by around 2.30 p.m. can be followed by light eating by 4.30 p.m. Around 6.30 to 7.30 p.m. you can ideally have your dinner for the night. You can retire for the day by around 10 p.m. to have comfortable sleep for eight hours.

In the evening as earlier stated metabolism slows down considerably and then food consumed should not be heavy. In fact by the time evening sets in a hormone called melatonin is secreted by the body which engages in the job of activities being folded up for the day. Energy requirement from then on till next day morning is at its lowest for the body. Therefore, evening eating can be spaced out by even up to two and a half or even three hours. Your body will be thankful to you for that.

14 EXERCISE IN
   MANAGING T2D

Exercise forms a very important factor in the self-management of diabetes. Type 2 Diabetes is a condition to be managed by the appropriate combination of diet, exercise and medication. While medication is not always a part of self-management of Type 2 Diabetes, diet and exercise are the two key factors central to any self-management programme aimed at managing it successfully. We have seen in the previous section how dietary changes have to be put in place as part of self management to derive optimum benefit in the successful management of Type 2 Diabetes. Once these two factors are successfully addressed almost all cases of Type 2 Diabetes can be managed very effectively with amazing outcome. Available indications justify that self-management accounts for about of eighty percent of diabetes management with medication taking care of only twenty percent. While this may vary in individual cases depending on age, constitution etc. of individuals, one is justified in maintaining that self-management is indeed the most important aspect of Type 2 Diabetes management. Self-management essentially comprises dietary changes and appropriate physical activity with other aspects like keeping regular sleeping hours and regularity with regard to other activities forming a minor yet significant part. Let us take a look at exercise in some detail now.

In persons not fully under the grip of Type 2 Diabetes or non-diabetics and pre-diabetics, exercise plays a very crucial role in that regular exercise can ensure that they are not led to being slaves to the condition of being Type 2 Diabetics. Exercise helps keep the general health of the body by improving the functioning of the heart, maintaining blood vessels in good condition and by improving good cholesterol content and lowering bad cholesterol content. Apart from this, it burns blood glucose directly and improves insulin functioning all at one go. All these factors have an aggregate effect of dragging one away from the unwelcome prospect of developing Type 2 Diabetes.

In the case of persons with Type 2 Diabetes also exercise forms one of the most important factors in managing it satisfactorily. Dieting, exercise and medication are the three pillars on which a concrete platform for management of Type 2 Diabetes is to be created. With appropriate dieting, as explained in the previous section, one can ensure that calorie intake by way of food is almost equal to the energy used by the body in which case theoretically blood glucose level should not be getting unduly disturbed. There will not be any glucose left unutilized and there will not be then any fat formation or resultant weight gain either. In such a scenario, theoretically again, there is no need for exercise as part of a regimen aimed at managing Type 2 Diabetes. Nor is there any case for any medication to manage Type 2 Diabetes.

In reality, however, this is seldom achieved in practice. In line with the habits developed as part of living in the modern world, one tends to add a little extra here and a little extra there while consuming food thus deviating from laid down dietary plans. This could be as part of eating out or part of the eating attendant to social and official gatherings or as part of the forced requirement while on travel and so on. Excess calorie intake thus coming in due to whatever reason can be prevented from interfering with one's management of Type 2 Diabetes by settling for an appropriate exercise programme aimed at burning out those extra calories. As a matter of fact, exercise has got very many beneficial effects other than helping maintaining blood sugar level in a healthy range. However an appropriate combination of dieting and exercising should ensure proper management of Type 2 Diabetes and can on their own ensure that blood glucose levels are maintained within permissible levels in most cases.

Medication theoretically needs to be resorted to only in cases where the combination of dietary changes and exercise fails to address the need to maintain blood sugar level in the permissible band on a continuous basis. Without going into more details one can safely maintain that dieting, exercising and taking medicines in that order are the three important factors in the successful management of Type 2 Diabetes. That is to say dietary changes or proper intake of food—that is the right food taken in right manner at the right times—is the most important factor among the three. To put it simply the number one requirement or the first defence against Type 2 Diabetes is TO EAT RIGHT. Next comes exercise at achieving certain clear objectives. Thus RIGHT EXERCISE is the second most important factor in an effective Type 2 Diabetes control programme. Last among the three is taking the RIGHT MEDICATION.

As we have seen, eating right alone is generally sufficient to manage Type 2 Diabetes in a large number of cases. Correct exercise comes into play as an added tool to exercise control where the measure of blood glucose reduction achieved through dieting is not adequate. This can be due to occasional or continuous deviation from correct eating. It can as well be due to the necessity in a case where the blood glucose level is out of control to the extent that it can not be addressed by dietary changes alone even if the eating is right in all respects. Extending it further, if right eating and combining it with right exercising fail to control blood sugar levels adequately or to the desired levels, medicines come into the frame for achieving that objective. Having taken a fairly detailed look at eating right, let us now take a close look at exercising right.

So here we go.

Exercise plays a very important role not just in the management of Type 2 Diabetes but in the proper maintenance of general health. All the same an exercise programme should not be followed indiscriminately. Exercise generally can be considered as voluntary physical activity pursued for its own sake with the objective of achieving specific goals which need not be related to health at all like in the case of getting prepared for some sport or athletic activity. While exercise no doubt is important in the management of Type 2 Diabetes, one should take note of the fact that physical activity of all kinds will contribute to healthy management of Type 2 Diabetes. The activity can be voluntary or involuntary. That is to say physical activity in relation to management of Type 2 Diabetes need not necessarily be in the nature of exercise but can well be routine physical activity as well. As a first step in this direction one should attempt enhancing the scope of involuntary activities as that would go a long way in achieving excellent results in the management of Type 2 Diabetes.

As a case in point while doing the painting, colour washing and routine maintenance work in my house I used to continuously engage in activities like shifting of furniture items, cupboards etc. to facilitate proper colour washing of the walls, cleaning of floors etc. The house I was staying in then was a sprawling 3000 square feet villa spread over three floors. Cleaning up the floors, stair way rails, windows etc. was also sparingly done by me partly by way of assisting the workers involved and partly by way of supervising the execution of the work. The point is I was fully involved in the work and thoroughly enjoyed the activity. Putting fixtures and furniture items back in place on completion of work and very often rearranging the items and bits of work like that ensured that I was physically very much enjoyably involved with the goings on. Never for a moment did I feel tired or bored during the ten week period I was on this job during my spare time after regular office work. On week ends and holidays I was almost fully immersed in this work.

Shortly after completion of the maintenance work mentioned above I was also due to check my HbA1C level. When checked this time it showed a decline to just below 6 from the earlier 7 plus level. This was indeed a bonus as far as my diabetic management was concerned. The only factor that has brought about this improvement was my engaging in physical activity while the home maintenance work was on. And this was enjoyable work and more importantly involuntary physical activity. Not that I undertook the activity to bring down my average blood glucose level but that the improvement in blood glucose level was a fall out of my involuntary work which was almost in the nature of a routine. But it paid handsome dividends in the context of management of my Type 2 Diabetes. The point is rather than pursue exercise as something you are forced to do, building physical activity into our routine will go a long way in achieving results we want to achieve through exercise. This will not diminish your enjoyment also since exercise for the sake of doing it is conceived as boring by great many individuals. And rightly so.

Exercise is only one component of physical activity. Exercise generally refers to structured and planned body movement pursued with a certain objective like reducing weight or improving mobility or improving clinical conditions like hypertension or similar conditions. Physical activity also involves unstructured activities like partaking in household work, commuting to office or going by foot for shopping, movements while moving about in one's work place and so on and so forth. These movements are not structured for deriving any physical benefits and they are carried out not as part of any conscious decision to engaging in physical activities. From the stand point of maintaining good control over blood sugar, both activities—structured activities like exercise and unstructured activities involving body movements off and on practiced as a matter of routine—are equally important. Engaging in routine activities if structured to an extent can create a situation where one can dispense with the need to engage in any physical activity that can be labeled as exercise as such. One's effort should be aimed at enhancing the scope of physical activity to such an extent that all possible scope for physical activity is exploited to the hilt in our routine living. Economising on physical effort which has unfortunately become an essential feature of modern living should be as a concept discarded for good.

In this context one may be reminded of the definition of Type 2 Diabetes in Ayurveda. Ayurveda maintains that one has a propensity to develop diabetes—what it calls *madhumeha*—when one feels like walking while wanting to run, one feels like sitting while wanting to walk, one feels like lying down while wanting to sit, and one feels like sleeping while wanting to lie down in the ordinary course of one's daily activities. Reversing this condition requires of one to simply keeping awake while wanting to sleep during day time, keeping a sitting posture while wanting to lie down, to keep standing while wanting to sit and to keep walking while wanting to sit down and rest on account of feeling tired or feeling that you are not equal to the task. Engaging in physical activity will help burn blood glucose directly and bring blood glucose level from higher to normal level. Thus attempting to walk while wanting to sit and similar deliberate physical engagements will have a very substantial beneficial impact on the overall management of Type 2 Diabetes. These actions when pursued will also have the feature that in effect one is reversing the causative factors that contributed to the development of Type 2 Diabetes in the first place. That is to say, if one was to have properly engaged in physical activities to the extent required and in tune with one's food intake in the past, in all probability one would not have turned Type 2 Diabetic. Now when physical activity is very deliberately taken up it will have the effect of slowly but surely beginning to reverse the causative factors that contributed to the present condition. When one begins to walk instead of standing and to walk briskly instead of walking slowly that very change will bring about health benefits and functional efficiency all of a sudden without any risk or harm. One can definitely practice this and derive benefits by parking the car at a fair distance away from where one wants to go and footing down the distance in between. One can try and practice using stairs instead of lift if not for going up at least for coming down a few floors to begin with. While in an escalator one can still climb a few steps. One can usefully engage in household chores without keeping an eye on saving effort and do things like climbing to the room upstairs whenever possible by taking up one mission at a time rather than clubbing all your activities upstairs in one go. One can wash one's vehicle once in a while or at least clean up the interiors and exteriors using a damp cloth. One can engage in gardening almost endlessly and can have the immense satisfaction that is one's when instrumental in two flowers blooming in place of only one earlier. The possibilities are endless if only you look out for the opportunities.

Then there are a lot of technical jargons associated with exercise which are held as capable of putting off one who is stepping into the terrain hesitantly. Terms like aerobic exercise, resistance exercise, isotonic exercise and a lot of similar jargons have made pure and simple physical activity look like a difficult proposition to take up. Then there are the medically contributed issues like contra indications for certain type of exercises for certain type of persons. All these and similar literature and thinking about exercise have had a cumulative effect of something like pouring cold water over a Type 2 Diabetic desirous of taking up exercise in a serious manner.

In the context of managing Type 2 Diabetes efficiently in most cases—actually almost all cases— brisk walking would serve the purpose completely as far as exercising for management of the condition is concerned. It is easy to perform, enjoyable and one can do it just about every where and at about any point of time. It does not require the support of any equipment either. Experiments have indicated that brisk walking for about thirty minutes brings down blood glucose level by at least ten points directly and immediately.

Apart from this walking has got beneficial effect on one's feeling level as well. It brings about overall improvement in one's biochemical processes and helps improve social dynamics as well. Walking, among other things, also helps in bringing about weight reduction and also in maintaining body weight at healthy levels continuously.

Even though compared to activities like swimming, riding, trekking etc. walking seems to be a docile affair, the fact remains that it is proved to be the best available exercise for various reasons. First, unlike playing tennis or riding or rowing, walking does not require one to have any special skills for engaging in it. It is something one is used to doing from early childhood. Secondly, it is not a taxing or demanding physical activity. Thirdly, it can be practiced by anyone anywhere and at any point of time. While these features make walking an eminently acceptable proposition as a physical activity that can be recommended for practice by diabetics, the most important reason for advocating this is not any of these. It is in fact the adequacy of walking as an activity to maintain overall health including efficient management of Type 2 Diabetes. As a physical activity walking is in fact a necessary and sufficient physical activity required to be carried out for one to have any meaningful control over Type 2 Diabetes.

As a matter of fact, decent control over blood sugar levels can be achieved by engaging in about thirty minutes of walking five days a week. While doing it every day regularly is always good, doing it five days in a week has been shown to have the required benefits for a diabetic. By doing so whatever control can be achieved through physical activity is seen substantially achieved. Out of thirty minutes of walking about twenty minutes should be utilized for brisk walking with about five minutes each or so devoted to warming up initially and gradually signing off towards a close. Walking for more than this in one go at a time is seen only to help burn calories without any direct benefit in the management of Type 2 Diabetes and here a word of caution also is necessary. Since Type 2 Diabetics usually follow strict dieting, walking for more than this unless supplemented by correspondingly higher food intake can bring in fatigue and tiredness. That is to say, it will only make one tired if one is following one's dietary regulations correctly. In case possible walking spread over two sessions can be thought of with one session in the morning and the second session in the evening. However one should ensure that walking per session is not allowed to go beyond 25 to thirty minutes.

While walking one should take certain precautions in case one is already taking insulin shots or certain category of medicines for Type 2 Diabetes. First, walking should be engaged in only when your blood glucose level is above 100. If on medicines and if your blood glucose level is below 100 or above 250 mg/dL, it is desirable not to undertake any form of exercise including walking. 100 to 250 mg/dL is generally considered the safe range of blood glucose level to be maintained for pursuing exercise by a Type 2 Diabetic. While walking can be engaged in even if blood glucose level is in the vicinity of 250, doing it when blood glucose is below 100 can cause hypoglycemia or fall in blood sugar to dangerously low levels. One should always be aware of this. Keeping some sugar or candies on one's person will be beneficial in this regard for use in the case of an emergency.

Apart from helping reduce blood glucose level walking is beneficial for increasing HDL or what is referred to as good cholesterol. Again, walking in the sun is even more beneficial since that way one gets to gain a lot of vitamin D as well which is otherwise very difficult to come by. Vitamin D is also seen to have beneficial impact on maintenance of blood glucose in the permissible range. Walking in the same manner in the same location can however turn out to be boring when it is regularly done. To surmount this problem and add variety to your walking, different routes can be chosen for walking each day of the week. Walking in the company of others regularly is seen to impart some sort of an element of compulsion to its performance on a regular basis. This can also be attempted. The idea is that one should make it a point to walk briskly for about twenty minutes on at least five days in a week positively without fail. Do ensure that this is carried out in rain and sunshine alike. Winter or summer, this should be regularly done. Tendency to hide behind excuses like rain, lack of enough time, travel and so on should not be resorted to for failing in undertaking this regular walk. As a physical activity beneficial to your maintaining good health and maintaining your blood glucose levels correctly, this is not asking for more and one should realize it before even thinking to call off one's walking under one pretext or other. As pointed out earlier, to start with, this is adequate for one to maintain his blood glucose levels under reasonably good control. As you gain greater control over your blood glucose and as you start enjoying walking, you can add more and more activities to your schedule if you like it that way. Or, if you want to stick to your original routine, keep it that way. Whatever your choice, do ensure that walking you do regularly.

While walking one should also try to take snacks or light refreshments after one finishes walking and not before one starts to walk. This way it works better. Some persons go for walk after eating, but this is not recommended. A light stroll after dinner, if one has been used to doing it, is fine but this is not recommended to be taken up afresh from the perspective of having a beneficial impact on one's blood sugar control programme.

15 MEDICATION

Medication is the third arm of management of Type 2 Diabetes. One has to necessarily take medicines for keeping blood sugar in the normal range if and only if dietary changes and exercise together fail to accomplish that task. Medication usually given for controlling Type 2 Diabetes and thus forming part of its management can be classified broadly into three categories. The first category of medicines aim improvement of the insulin efficiency of the system in charge of metabolism. In a manner of speaking, these attempt to squeeze more insulin out of the pancreas with a view to handling the carbohydrate intake better. The second category of medicines inhibits release of glucose reserve from the liver and thus ensures that blood glucose levels are not allowed to go up in an uncontrolled manner. This category of medicines also aid weight reduction to an extent thus making the body make better use of available insulin. A third category of medicines slows down absorption of glucose from the intestine.

These three categories of medicines perform distinctly different functions. A combination of these three categories that works for a given Type 2 Diabetic can be decided on only after a trial and error involving administration of these medicines in combination over a period of time. During this period of trial and error a medical practitioner will be assessing the efficacy of the combination on a given individual. During this period, based on the observed behavior of blood glucose level changes in the individual, changes will be made in the exact combination and measure of the three categories of medicine. In case the combination of drugs fail to have blood sugar maintained within the desirable levels, one may be advised to go in for insulin injections as well. There is a school of thought among medical practitioners who maintain that insulin should form part of the first level of defence in the management of Type 2 Diabetes. Doctors belonging to this school of thought tend to put the Type 2 Diabetics on insulin straightaway with the combination of the three category of drugs mentioned also forming part of the medication package. The question whether insulin is to be started and if to be started when to start is better left to the physician. Likewise prescription of medicines including the combination and quantity of each is better left to the medical practitioner. However, there are certain important points one should give special attention to.

While a medical practitioner will prescribe the tablets for you, you are entitled to and must definitely know which medicine you are taking for what. Persons with Type 2 Diabetes are generally given tablets other than those that are instrumental in bringing the blood glucose level down. These include medicines for proper maintenance of blood pressure and in certain cases tablets aimed at preventing damage to kidneys and pre-empting cardiovascular complications. More often than not multivitamin tablets are required to be taken as a matter of routine. A person taking these tablets should certainly know which tablet is taken for what. As for tablets taken for purposes other than bringing down blood sugar level, one must well remember that these are given as a matter of precaution. The precaution is taken since a Type 2 Diabetic is susceptible to contracting various complicated conditions if blood sugar levels are not maintained within the permissible limits. Hence these tablets are better advised to be taken, and should be taken for as long as required by one's physician.

The point to be noted very clearly at this point is that intake of medicines including insulin injection if any to an extent forms part of the self management of Type 2 Diabetes. Again, it must be emphasized that all matters related to administration of medicine is best left to the medical practitioner. But there are instances when a person should know when to take and when not to take a medicine directed at controlling blood sugar. For example, medicines are given to suit a typical day in the life of a Type 2 Diabetic. In actual situation on a day there could be deviations from the normal assumed routine for any one. On these days one should keep a careful watch over the medicines taken. When you have food intake as per a given schedule, and when your physical activity in a day is as envisaged to be ideal, you will need to take insulin injection and blood sugar controlling medicines as prescribed. This will not be the best way to go about taking medicines on a day when there is change in dietary intake or physical activity. Continuing with one's prescribed medicines when you have not eaten as per your schedule or when you have performed additional physical work can result in blood sugar level falling below the permissible level. Walking an extra mile or two or doing some physical activity which is not part of the normal routine can create such a situation. Under such circumstances there is a possibility of hypoglycemia setting in with undesirable consequences. One should be aware of conditions attendant to Type 2 Diabetes in order to avoid such situations. To this extent medication also falls in the territory of efficient self management of the condition.

While doctors are the best judges of such situations, when such situations do occur a doctor's advice may not readily be available. Efficient self management of Type 2 Diabetes calls for reducing the intake of blood sugar lowering medicines in such conditions if not deciding to dispense with taking medicines for an interval of time till your doctor is able to guide you correctly. As one can easily see, taking medication to lower blood glucose when one's blood glucose level is already low can be disastrous. The possible resultant hyperglycemia or increase in blood sugar level above the permissible limit will be only a temporary feature. One should well remember that temporary spike in blood glucose level is preferred to a fall in blood sugar below the minimum required level. In the language of medicine it is stated as hyperglycemia being preferred to hypoglycemia. Blood glucose level spiking once in a while is not a fraction as harmful as it falling to dangerously low levels. Testing one's blood glucose level on occasions like this is to be resorted to. Testing is now a days very easy and can be swiftly done using an ordinary blood glucose measuring meter. On ascertaining the actual blood sugar level a view can be taken by the person himself immediately perhaps in the nature of a first aid. Being familiar with tips like this can make a critical difference at times, and to this extent medication also needs to be thought of as part of self management. Another useful tip one should go by is to carry always glucose, food and drinking water while driving or undertaking long distance journey. Keep checking blood sugar level if you are on insulin and make sure that you occupy driver's seat only when your blood glucose level is within the normal range.

Self management aspect of medication comes into play during certain occasions whether one likes it or not. As a case in point, when you are undertaking long distance travel your dietary and physical activity schedules may not be capable of being correctly implemented. When you are faced with a situation where you can not have food as planned—as you would like to have it in terms of nature, quantity or timing— there is a case for taking a relook at taking the blood sugar lowering medicines. Or for that matter the insulin injection you are required to take is to be reviewed. In the case of certain insulins, you are required to take adequate food within about fifteen to twenty minutes of taking the insulin shot. When you are taking insulin at a scheduled time without being in a position to take food as required, you have a problem on your hand.

While on such insulin you can not—YOU CAN NOT—cut down on your normal intake of food. If you do that you are in all probability going to have your blood glucose fall to alarmingly low level. In situations like this, you have to take a call on whether or not to take the insulin shot. Your ability to self manage comes into play here. Likewise when you are more than ordinarily active physically on a day for whatever reason, there is a case for decreasing insulin intake and reducing blood sugar lowering medicines. Or to tide over the situation you have to take the call on how much food intake should be there to offset the effect of your activity on blood glucose level. The carbohydrate intake is to be increased or medical intervention needs to be reduced in such a situation. Here also, your self management skill is called upon to act in an appropriate manner. The dynamic balance among diet, physical activity and medication is to be correctly maintained for the proper management of blood sugar levels. Any change in one area needs to be set off by appropriate adjustments in the level of the other two. Here self management is of critical significance.

While on medication blood glucose levels should be frequently monitored including HbA1C level every three months. What you can not know or measure you can not monitor. So blood glucose level should be measured at different points of time of the day rather frequently till the HbA1C level is around six to seven on a sustainable basis. Based on the regular blood sugar level readings you take frequently, you will have to adjust your diet, level of physical activity and even insulin intake till such time you are out of the clutches of Type 2 Diabetes. Care should however be taken to ensure that your insulin intake is only adjusted only downwards and not upwards. That is to say your insulin intake should never go beyond the level indicated by your physician. This is very important.

Properly managed as you move on, with effective self management interventions, you should be able to bring down dependence on medicines to a large extent. However, if one is on medication all aspects of taking medicines should be left to your physician. The point to be noted is to get all your doubts clarified with the medical practitioner and that you should most certainly be aware of which medicines are being taken with the expected purpose of each medicine. The importance of this can not be and should not be overlooked.

16 SUMMING IT UP

Type 2 Diabetes is the most common form of diabetes, and the incidence of this is increasing at an alarming rate. In part this is held to be on account of the genetic predisposition of people of certain ethnic features. Indians figure prominently in this list of people likely to be affected by Type 2 Diabetes. Whatever be the arguments for and against this, one thing is certain—Type 2 Diabetes is a condition predominantly brought about by following certain life style which is amenable to correction. Type 2 Diabetes is not to be treated as an illness in the sense that there is no cure for this. As we have heard many say, one has to live with diabetes once one is affected by it. In other words, it can not be cured, but can only be managed. But we have been discussing how one can successfully get over this condition on a sustainable basis and continue to lead a very normal life in all probability without any medicinal aid.

From whatever has been discussed so far, one should have got a fairly good idea of how Type 2 Diabetes would have set in in the first place. Cure for this, we do not have as yet, but managing it we certainly can. Forming part of managing it is the intake of appropriate drugs as prescribed by the physician. But managing for the most part is a function to be performed by the affected person himself. That is to say self management forms the most important aspect of managing diabetes. In fact self management should aim at controlling the condition initially and then progress to managing it effectively. If one tries a little hard enough, one can not just manage Type 2 Diabetes but can successfully reverse it.

Controlling blood sugar is to be brought about first by monitoring blood glucose levels frequently at irregular times followed by HbA1C test every three to four months. Secondly it is to be achieved by bringing about suitable life style changes as discussed earlier along with appropriate clinical support wherever necessary. Monitoring blood glucose levels frequently at irregular times is important till such time one gets a measure of success in managing the condition effectively. It is not enough if one checks one's blood glucose levels every week looking only at fasting blood sugar level. One has to necessarily monitor fasting blood glucose followed by the blood sugar readings after taking breakfast, then after lunch and then post dinner and before going to bed not necessarily on the same day but spread over different days. Once in a while one has to go in for random checking of blood sugar as well. Again, once in a while all the above readings have to be taken on a given day just to get an idea of the behavior and pattern one's blood sugar is following. In each individual the pattern followed is found to be different. That is the reason why continuous normal fasting blood sugar does not necessarily mean that one's overall blood sugar level is within permissible levels. This is a mistake usually done. While visiting physician one always goes in for the fasting blood sugar level and sometimes the level after two hours of having breakfast. With normal readings for these two the HbA1C level is seen to be high on many occasions. This is so because there could probably be a tendency for blood sugar to go up well after the time the two readings are taken. This would also be a pattern in respect of a person resulting in A1C test showing spiked average blood glucose. Just to get an idea of when one's blood sugar levels normally peak and normally reach its lowest level for an individual, this frequent check is essential and is an indispensible part of successful management of Type 2 Diabetes. Then again, one has to check the HbA1C levels every three to four months so as to take on hand fresh corrective action if this level is above 7 per cent,

Appropriate life style changes have to be brought in next. This includes both dietary changes and changes related to physical activity. Dietary changes are to be brought about in such a manner to have the erratic or deviant eating corrected to the required extent. For example, if fasting blood sugar is say 120 mg/dL, then one should change the content and reduce the quantity of food being taken at dinner. May be one can replace rice with wheat or go low on bread and add more vegetables, cut down or change the fruit taken post dinner or avoid that dessert or glass of milk after dinner or before going to bed. In a similar way take a critical look at the diet that one has had before one had seen a higher than permissible blood glucose level, and bring in the required changes in the nature and quantity of food taken prior to the erratic reading. Same applies for physical activity as well. A more than normal level in blood glucose to the extent of 10 to 15 points can be ordinarily offset by walking for about twenty minutes or a half hour by way of additional physical output.

Appropriate clinical support comprises support by way of investigative and diagnostic inputs. These include checking of the physical parameters with regard to functioning of the heart, nerves, teeth and eyes and also checking of blood for getting the lipid profile, creatine levels etc., and periodic checking of blood pressure and body weight. Once the diagnostic results are in place, appropriate drugs and / or insulin may have to be prescribed in relation to the results keeping in view one's age. This is how one's blood glucose levels have to be kept monitored and brought under control along with other complementary health parameters.

Let a new beginning be made here and now to keep your blood glucose level in the normal range. Today is the first day in the rest of your life. Let a new beginning be made now itself. The past is over and the future is just beginning. Strive to achieve normal blood sugar levels on a sustainable basis from now on.

Good Luck.

www.ingramcontent.com/pod-product-compliance
Lightning Source LLC
Chambersburg PA
CBHW050401290526
45786CB00003B/1074